RESOURCES

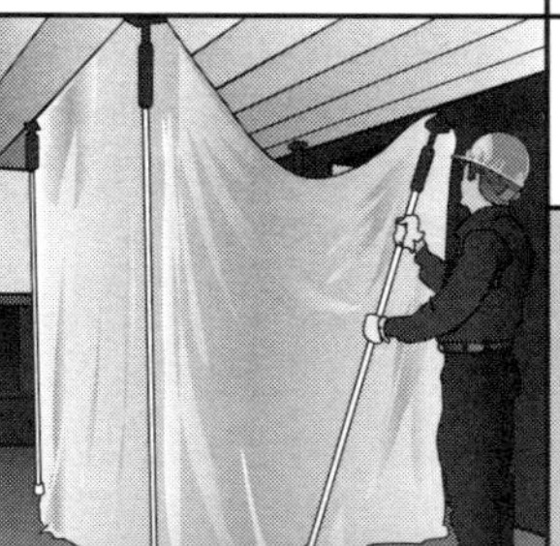

Planning, Design, and Construction OF HEALTH CARE FACILITIES

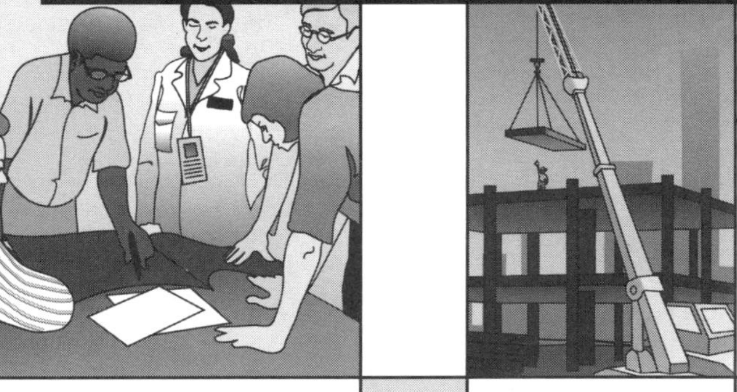

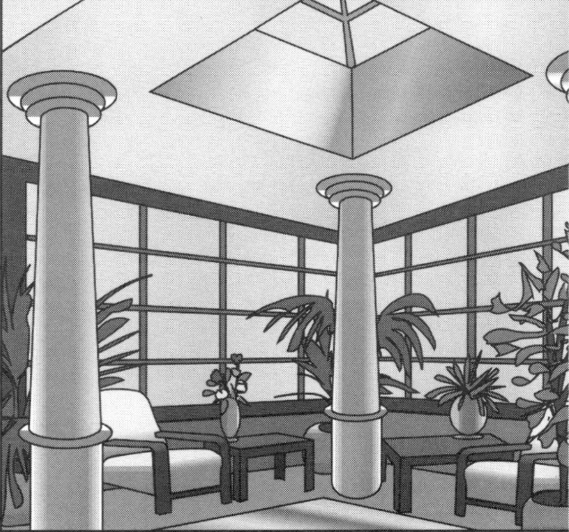

Improving Health Care Quality and Safety

Joint Commission Resources Mission

The mission of Joint Commission Resources is to continuously improve the safety and quality of care in the United States and in the international community through the provision of education and consultation services and international accreditation.

Joint Commission Resources educational programs and publications support, but are separate from, the accreditation activities of the Joint Commission. Attendees at Joint Commission Resources educational programs and purchasers of Joint Commission Resources publications receive no special consideration or treatment in, or confidential information about, the accreditation process.

The inclusion of an organization name, product, or service in a Joint Commission publication should not be construed as an endorsement of such organization, product, or service, nor is failure to include an organization name, product, or service to be construed as disapproval.

This publication is designed to provide accurate and authoritative information in regard to the subject matter covered. Every attempt has been made to ensure accuracy at the time of publication; however, please note that laws, regulations, and standards are subject to change. Please also note that some of the examples in this publication are specific to the laws and regulations of the locality of the facility. The information and examples in this publication are provided with the understanding that the publisher is not engaged in providing medical, legal, or other professional advice. If any such assistance is desired, the services of a competent professional person should be sought.

Joint Commission Resources, Inc. (JCR), a not-for-profit affiliate of the Joint Commission on Accreditation of Healthcare Organizations (Joint Commission), has been designated by the Joint Commission to publish publications and multimedia products. JCR reproduces and distributes these materials under license from the Joint Commission.

Printed in the U.S.A. 5 4 3 2 1

ISBN: 0-86688-952-3

LCCN: 2005932641

For more information about Joint Commission Resources, please visit http://www.jcrinc.com.

Senior Editor:
Kristine M. Miller, M.F.A.

Project Manager:
Christine Wyllie

Manager, Publications:
Diane Bell

Production Manager:
Johanna Harris

Associate Director:
Cecily Pew

Executive Director:
Catherine Chopp Hinckley, Ph.D.

Joint Commission Reviewers:
George Mills, F.A.S.H.E, C.H.F.M, C.E.M, *Associate Director, Standards Interpretation Group*

Jerry Gervais, C.H.F.M, C.H.S.P, *Associate Director, Standards Interpretation Group*

Megan Sawchuk, M.T., *Associate Director, Standards Interpretation Group*

John Fishbeck, R.A., *Associate Project Director, Standards Interpretation Group*

Darryl S. Rich, Pharm.D., M.B.A., F.A.S.H.P. *Field Representative*

Other Expert Reviewers:
Kristi Ennis, A.I.A., *Sustainable Design Director, Senior Associate, Boulder Associates, Inc., Architecture + Interior Design, Boulder, CO*

David K. Samples, *Facilities Engineer & Construction, Facilities Management Department, Elmhurst Memorial Healthcare, Elmhurst, IL*

Requests for permission to make copies of any part of this work should be mailed to

Permissions Editor
Department of Publications
Joint Commission Resources
One Renaissance Boulevard
Oakbrook Terrace, Illinois 60181
permissions@jcrinc.com

TABLE OF CONTENTS

INTRODUCTION

CREATING SOMETHING FROM NOTHING is an awesome task. It requires forethought, creativity, commitment, and enthusiasm. If this "something" is as large as a new building or a renovated space, it also requires planning, resources, education, and communication. The planning, design, and construction process can be daunting if health care organizations do not have the appropriate tools, personnel, and commitment for the task. Multidisciplinary collaboration must occur throughout all stages of the process, and patients, staff, and the community should play an integral role.

The purpose of this publication is to help health care organization leaders, environment of care professionals, and other health care organization staff members successfully navigate the planning, design, and construction process. While the scope of this publication does not allow for detailed examination of every aspect of the process, it does offer some guidelines organizations can use in planning and implementation.

The Six Phases of the Building Process

Any time an organization embarks on a large project, it can be helpful to reduce that project to small, easy-to-manage parts. With that in mind, most building projects can be organized into six distinct phases:

1. ***Planning.*** This includes blue-sky considerations, master planning, and predesign efforts
2. ***Schematic design.*** This involves drawing a rough outline of the project, including preliminary room layout, structure, and scope
3. ***Design and development.*** This involves adding details to the design, including fixtures, furniture location, and decor
4. ***Construction documents.*** This involves converting all aspects of the design into a template from which contractors can estimate costs, identify issues, and plan construction activities. At this point organizations will discuss contract conditions, including general conditions and those specific to the project.
5. ***Construction.*** This is the process in which the building or facility is actually built
6. ***Commissioning.*** Before taking ownership of the building, project, or renovation, organizations must make sure all specifications are met, and all systems, components, equipment, and so forth are fully operational. Commissioning encompasses these activities.

Although some of these phases can overlap, they are usually implemented sequentially. They provide a framework for the building process; however, some degree of variation is common on almost every building project.

Content of the Book

The chapters within this publication are organized to follow the previously mentioned phases. Chapters One and Two discuss issues and actions related to planning. Chapter One looks at the variety of considerations organizations should keep in mind when conceptualizing the building and building process. Chapter Two discusses more concrete steps, such as team selection, programming, scheduling, communication, and budgeting.

Chapter Three takes a focused look at the Joint Commission's requirements regarding planning, design, and construction. Areas such as safety, security, emergency management, infection control, and fire safety are discussed. The chapter also provides information on the Joint Commission's requirements regarding the proactive risk assessment process and interim life safety measures.

Chapter Four moves past the planning phase and examines the schematic design, design development, construction documents, and construction phases. It provides general information on what organizations can expect during these phases and offers suggestions to ensure effective communication and implementation of risk-reduction strategies throughout the different phases.

The final chapter, Chapter Five, briefly discusses the commissioning process. While not difficult conceptually, this process can be challenging for organizations if they do not prepare for it early. The chapter offers some tips and strategies to successfully commission a new or renovated building.

The two appendixes take a closer look at areas that require special design considerations: the laboratory and pharmacy. Meeting regulations, ensuring proper ventilation, and enhancing patient and staff safety are paramount in these areas.

Although every construction project will be different, organizations can keep certain concepts in mind throughout building efforts. Those organizations that plan, communicate, respond to input, and address the needs and concerns of patients and staff can successfully navigate the building process. After completing the project, organizations should be proud of their accomplishments and know that their hard work, diligence, and enthusiasm resulted in creating a dynamic, focused, and safe environment.

Acknowledgements

A work of this scope requires a concerted team effort. This volume, which we hope you find to be as useful as it is practical, could not have been created without such a team. We are deeply indebted to our writer, Kathleen B. Vega, for her hours of research, interviewing, and writing; her careful attention to detail; and her consummate professionalism.

We wish to acknowledge the outstanding contribution to the completion of this book by our Joint Commission and outside expert reviewers (see the masthead on page ii).

The writer wishes to thank the following individuals, who gave freely of their time and expertise to provide information and resources:

- R. Stephen Bolshazy, F.H.F.I., health care facility, medical equipment planning, and project management consultant, located in Escondido, California
- Therese Bovee-McKelvey, R.N., M.N., C.O.H.N.-S., occupational health services manager for Seattle Children's Hospital & Regional Medical Center, located in Seattle, Washington
- Kristi Ennis, A.I.A., L.E.E.D. Accredited Professional, senior associate for Boulder Associates, Inc., located in Boulder, Colorado
- Jerry Gervais, C.H.F.M, C.H.S.P., associate director for the Standards Interpretation Group, Division of Accreditation Operations at the Joint Commission, located in Oakbrook Terrace, Illinois
- Tom Gormley, vice president of HCA Healthcare Corp., located in Nashville, Tennessee
- Robin Guenther, A.I.A., president of Guenther 5 Architects, located in New York City
- Bruce R. Harrison, M.S., R.Ph., B.C.O.P., clinical pharmacy specialist for the Veterans Affairs Medical Center, located in St. Louis
- James Jorgenson, M.S., R.Ph., director of pharmacy services for University of Utah Hospitals and Clinics, located in Salt Lake City
- Karen Lambert, M.S., president of Advocate Good Shepherd Hospital, located in Barrington, Illinois
- Debra J. Levin, B.S.D., M.A.M., president of the Center for Health Design, located in Concord, California
- Jain Malkin, president of Jain Malkin Inc., located in San Diego, California
- George Mills, F.A.S.H.E, C.H.F.M, C.E.M, associated director for the Standards Interpretation Group, Division of Accreditation Operations at the Joint Commission, located in Oakbrook Terrace, Illinois
- William Morgan, S.A.S.H.E. C.H.F.M., manager of plant operations and facility engineering for Saint Alphonsus Regional Medical Center, located in Boise, Idaho
- Karen Mortland, A.I.A. M.T.(A.S.C.P.), president of Mortland Planning & Design, Inc., located in Chicora, Pennsylvania
- Roseanne Niese, R.N., B.S.N., director of emergency, intensive care & nursing resource services for Advocate Good Shepherd Hospital, located in Barrington, Illinois
- Leo Old, P.E., C.I.H., senior consultant for Smith Seckman Reid, Inc., located in Memphis, Tennessee
- Allison Prehn, architecture student at Texas A&M School of Architecture, located in College Station, Texas
- John Reeve, principal and CEO of Christner Inc., located in St. Louis
- John Reiling, M.A., M.B.A., president/chief executive officer for St. Joseph's Hospital, located in West Bend, Wisconsin
- Sue Reinoehl, vice president of business development for Bronson Healthcare Group, Inc., located in Kalamazoo, Michigan
- David K. Samples, facilities engineer for Elmhurst Memorial Healthcare, located in Elmhurst, Illinois
- Frank Sardone, president and CEO of Bronson Healthcare Group, Inc., located in Kalamazoo, Michigan
- Annemarie Schmocker, R.N., B.S.N., infection control practitioner for Elmhurst Memorial Healthcare, located in Elmhurst, Illinois
- Enrique Unanue, A.I.A., N.C.A.R.B., A.C.H.A. deputy director of the Illinois Department of Public Health, located in Springfield, Illinois
- Tom Van Landingham, associate, senior project manager for Christner, Inc., located in St. Louis

CHAPTER ONE:

Considerations for Building Health Care Facilities

A CONSTRUCTION BOOM IS UNDERWAY in health care, with a significant number of hospital projects in progress, not to mention construction projects in long term care, behavioral health care, and ambulatory care facilities.[1] Upgrade and repair projects jumped nearly 30% in the late 1990s and show no signs of slowing.[2] In 2004, hospitals across the country spent more than $16 billion for construction, and this number is predicted to increase to more than $20 billion by 2010.[3] These figures reveal one of the largest health care building booms in U.S. history, rivaling the period immediately following World War II.

The Effects of Hill-Burton

In 1946 Congress passed the Hospital Survey and Construction Act, more widely known as the Hill-Burton Act after its two sponsoring senators. The law was designed to provide federal grants to modernize existing hospitals that had become obsolete due to lack of capital investment throughout the period of the Great Depression and World War II. The law was also designed to provide funds to build new facilities in previously underserved areas. The Hill-Burton Act launched a nationwide hospital-building boom that resulted in new facilities all over the country, even in previously underserved rural communities.[4]

During the course of nearly 30 years, the Hill-Burton Act gave $4.6 billion in grant funds and $1.5 billion in loans to nearly 6,800 health care facilities in more than 4,000 communities.[5] While a great program in its time, one of its legacies includes many out-of-date hospital buildings that are in desperate need of replacement. Some of these facilities have not been updated, renovated, or remodeled since they were built. They are designed based on Hill-Burton standards and 50-year-old research and health care practices. Their infrastructure is crumbling, and their layout is out of date and ineffective at best. In some cases, the building itself fosters an environment where errors occur and safety is compromised. For example, noisy buildings with a cumbersome layout that limits communication can increase staff members' frustration and fatigue and thus affect their performance. This environment can be a hotbed for errors, as staff is tired, distracted, and not communicating effectively with each other.

While many health care facilities need to be replaced, building or renovating such facilities represents a significant capital expense for a health care organization. It is estimated that a new facility can cost an organization upwards of $1 million per patient bed. Moreover, given this huge expense, the final product will likely remain with an organization, its patients, and the community for years to come. The costs plus the lasting effects of building decisions make it critical that organizations think carefully before beginning a construction project.

Issues to Consider

When building a new facility, adding on to an existing facility, or renovating an existing facility, organizations should keep several considerations in mind. These considerations can affect the layout and design of the building; the cost of the building project; the facility's impact on patients, staff, and the community; and the organization's overall ability to provide safe, high-quality, and appropriate care and to adapt over time. Some issues organizations should consider include the following:

The safety and satisfaction of patients and staff. It takes a coordinated system, with all components of the system working together, to provide safe and effective health care. A health care organization's building is an integral part of that system. Recent evidence shows that the design of a health care building can not only improve patient safety, but also improve patient outcomes, decrease patient lengths of stay, reduce patient transfers, and increase patient and staff satisfaction.[3] Likewise, building designs can decrease employee frustration, improve job satisfaction, reduce absenteeism, and help organizations attract and retain staff. By incorporating a safe, patient-focused design that provides a healing environment, organizations can improve patient safety, patient outcomes, staff productivity, and overall patient and staff satisfaction

The needs of the community. Every organization serves a community, and the needs of that community will vary depending on the demographics of the population, the geographic location of the community, and the number of health care facilities available to treat the community. By assessing the needs of the community, organizations can determine the type of care that is necessary to meet those needs and the most effective design for that care. This assessment may reveal the need to downsize or specialize the care provided at a facility. It may also indicate areas that should receive more focused attention and space, such as having a larger emergency department or a more easily accessible outpatient facility.

Changes in technology. The technology and medical equipment available to health care organizations to provide high-quality, efficient, safe care is remarkably different than it was when many health care facilities were built, and organizations must consider how these changes will affect the design and layout of a new facility. Technology is changing at such a rapid pace that organizations must design facilities to be flexible so the facilities can efficiently incorporate current technology as well as future technology.

Environmental considerations. Siting, building materials, waste disposal, and water and energy usage are just some of the areas of building design and construction that can negatively impact the environment. By considering the environmental impact of project design elements, such as the type of building materials used, organizations can meet the needs of the community and protect the environment at the same time.

Efficiency. Remaining competitive and accommodating process redesign in health care is a major reason many organizations choose to build a replacement hospital.

By thinking about these issues prior to the design phase, organization leaders can have an understanding of the type of building and building process they want to have and whether it is feasible to accomplish their goals. The result of this "pre-analysis" can affect the type of design team chosen, the building materials used, the site of the facility, and many more factors.

This chapter provides a brief discussion of the previously mentioned considerations. The suggestions in this chapter will not apply to every organization, but they are offered here as a place to start thinking about issues.

Enhancing Patient and Staff Safety and Satisfaction

In its landmark report *To Err Is Human,* the Institute of Medicine estimated that between 44,000 and 98,000 people die each year as a result of medical errors. This is more than the number of people killed each year by motor vehicle accidents, breast cancer, or HIV/AIDS. The overwhelming majority of medical errors are not caused intentionally, but result from failures in the systems that support care. For example, poor communication, inadequate staffing, and lack of training can all lead to medical errors. An unsafe environment can also intensify and even foster the likelihood of errors in a health care organization. For example, lack of proper lighting, too much noise, overcrowding, and impure air are all environmental factors that can impede the safe delivery of care.

In a recent report entitled *The Role of the Physical Environment in the Hospital of the 21st Century: A Once-in-a Lifetime Opportunity,* Roger Ulrich and Craig Zimring argue that more than 600 credible studies show that a hospital's design can significantly improve patient safety, such as limiting health care–associated infections and decreasing medical errors.[3] The report also makes the case that facility design can impact staff performance, increase patient and staff satisfaction, and improve financial operations.

Just as there are proponents of using evidence-based medicine in health care delivery, Ulrich and Zimring and many others are proponents of using evidence-based design for health care construction. *Evidence-based design* (EBD) incorporates specific design principles that have been shown through comprehensive research studies to improve clinical and satisfaction outcomes for patients and staff.[6] The focus of EBD is to create facilities that enhance patient safety, help patients recover faster, and help staff perform better. (*See* Sidebar 1-1 on page 8). Following are some of the design principles included in EBD:

Build private rooms. By designing single-patient rooms that can accommodate a variety of equipment depending on the acuity of the patient, organizations can reap tremendous patient benefits, including the following:

- Reduce the spread of infection
- Decrease noise levels
- Increase patient and family privacy
- Foster patient and staff communication
- Decrease patient falls
- Reduce the number of patient transfers and associated medical errors
- Improve patient satisfaction
- Improve staff satisfaction

These rooms should have space for the patient and equipment and also for family members. Staff should also have space to move around the room without impacting the family or equipment space.

By designing patient rooms to accommodate a variety of equipment, organizations can reduce the need to transfer patients from one area to another for tests and procedures. These rooms, sometimes referred to as *variable acuity rooms,* can reduce the likelihood of patient and staff injury resulting from patient transfers, decrease the spread of infection, and reduce the likelihood of errors that occur as a result of transferring.[7] ■

Reduce noise levels. World Health Organization (WHO) guidelines suggest that background noise in hospital patient rooms should not exceed 35 dB, with nighttime peaks in wards not to exceed 40 dB. Unfortunately, many health care facilities have noise levels that are well above the recommended guidelines. Hospital noise comes from loud equipment, multiple voices speaking at once, overhead paging systems, and so forth. At the same time, environmental surfaces, such as floors, walls, and ceilings, are typically not sound absorbing—and can in fact amplify noise.[9] Prolonged exposure to environmental noise can increase stress, impact the ability to sleep, decrease tolerance for pain, and increase agitation. (*See* Sidebar 1-2 on page 9.) For staff, elevated noise levels can not only increase stress, but reduce concentration and limit communication. To improve noise levels, organizations should consider the following actions:

- Install sound-absorbing ceiling tiles or wall panels
- Carpet hallways to reduce the noise of moving equipment
- Decentralize nursing stations, where nurses, doctors, and other health care staff tend to congregate and talk
- Build single-patient rooms
- Mask noxious sounds with pleasant sounds, such as classical music or nature sounds
- Train staff to be aware of noise levels and teach them how to reduce noise, such as speaking more softly and turning off cell phones
- Eliminate overhead paging systems[10]

Incorporate nature into building design. Plants, fountains, waterfalls, gardens, and natural views can reduce patient and staff stress, improve morale, and lead to positive clinical outcomes. Access to nature can diminish negative emotions, such as fear and anger, and increase positive feelings. Individuals with access to nature in a health care facility have a higher tolerance for pain and tend to rely less on pain medications after treatment. Viewing nature or paintings of nature can result in physiological changes, including reduced blood pressure and heart activity. On the other hand, studies suggest that looking at built scenes that lack nature, such as rooms, buildings, and parking lots, can increase stress.[3]

Including gardens in the design of facilities can not only provide patients with calming views of nature, but can also reduce stress and improve outcomes through other mechanisms. Gardens can foster social support, provide opportunities to escape the stressful clinical environment, and allow patients and families to interact in a calm and restful setting. Long term care and behavioral health care patients can use gardens as a source for outdoor activity and exercise. Gardens also provide a place that staff, such as nurses and physicians, can go to take a break and recuperate from stress. Depending on the design, gardens can have additional positive environmental implications for a health care organization. For instance, gardens can provide increased shade for the facility and can reduce energy costs.[3] ■

SIDEBAR 1-1.
Center for Health Design

One of the leading proponents of evidence-based design is a nonprofit research and advocacy organization called the Center for Health Design. This organization helps health care organizations improve patient outcomes through the creative use of evidence-based design. The Center serves a network of more than 25,000 professionals worldwide and provides research, education, environmental standards, and technical assistance. The Center for Health Design was a main sponsor of the previously mentioned report by Roger Ulrich and Craig Zimring. The Center's Web site, www.healthdesign.org, provides valuable information and resources for those organizations planning and designing new or renovated facilities.[8]

Provide integrated and systemic wayfinding systems. Patients who have trouble finding their way in a health care facility may experience emotional stress from getting lost and worrying about arriving late for their appointments. Patients who are weak or disabled may suffer physically from going the wrong way and walking farther than needed. Families who enter a health care facility may already be stressed and distracted and getting lost will only exacerbate their situation. New staff may spend considerable time in their first days navigating a facility, and even existing staff can get lost if a facility's hallways all look the same.

SIDEBAR 1-2.
Noise Can Affect Even the Smallest Patients

Recent studies show that increased noise levels can have detrimental health effects on neonatal intensive care unit (NICU) patients. For example, infants exposed to higher noise levels require more oxygen support therapy. These infants also have elevated blood pressure, increased heart and respiration rates, and a lessened ability to sleep.[9]

In addition to the impact on patients and staff that poor wayfinding systems can have, organizations face a hidden financial impact as well. Every time a patient has to stop and ask a staff member for directions, the patient is pulling that staff member away from something else. A recent study revealed that staff in a 300-bed hospital spent 4,500 hours a year helping patients and visitors find their way. This led to an estimated cost of $220,000 per year, more than would be needed to install signs, maps, and information kiosks to help people find their own way.[11]

Organizations should consider wayfinding systems when planning a building project and throughout the design process. An effective wayfinding system is made up of carefully coordinated, consistent elements, including the following:

- Effective site and building layout
- Appropriate roadway and entranceway configuration
- Visible and easy-to-read exterior and interior signs
- Accessible directories
- Clear floor and room numbering
- Easy-to-read "You are here" signs and handheld maps
- Clearly marked emergency exit information
- Interior and exterior landmarks, such as unique design features
- Effective operational policies related to wayfinding, such as staff training and wayfinding system management

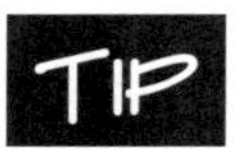

When designing a wayfinding system, organizations should make sure that signage is visible, easy to read, and quickly understandable. Organizations should consider putting directional signs at or before every major intersection or destination. Rooms should be numbered, and in some cases, changes in paint color or flooring material can be used to indicate a new department.[9] ■

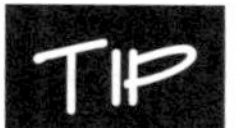

The design of a health care facility's entrance is critical for effective wayfinding. Entrances should be as obvious as possible. People driving by should be able to spot an entrance, as should people located in the parking area. Organizations can use environmental cues, such as canopies, pediments, flagpoles, and landscaping, to reinforce the presence of an entrance. Even details such as door material and hardware can indicate where a patient or visitor is supposed to enter. ■

Improve air quality. Ventilation and filtration not only make the air easier to breathe, but they also prevent the spread of airborne infection. Organizations should consider the most effective ways to keep the air "clean" to improve patient outcomes and staff productivity. Clean air can also reduce absenteeism and improve worker safety. Chapter Three addresses the importance of air quality in greater detail and provides specific tips that organizations can use to prevent the spread of infection and increase patient and staff safety.

Encourage hand washing. The most effective way to prevent the spread of infections in a health care facility is regular and thorough hand washing. Organizations should consider how to promote regular hand washing through facility design. There is support for the notion that numerous, conveniently located, alcohol-based hand-rub dispensers and hand-washing sinks can increase staff compliance with hand-washing protocols. In particular, putting hand-rub dispensers near the bedside usually improves compliance.[3] More information on how facility design affects infection control can be found in Chapter Three.

Incorporate light. Bright light during daytime hours, both natural and artificial, can help patients overcome depression, reduce agitation, and eventually sleep better. Bright light can also reduce lengths of stay and increase tolerance for pain.[9] Exposure to "daylighting," natural light through windows, can be especially helpful in improving patient satisfaction, reducing the need for pain killers, and decreasing lengths of stay. In addition, daylighting can reduce an organization's energy costs. (*See* the "Environmental Considerations" section beginning on page 21 in this chapter.)[1] Some ways to effectively incorporate bright light or daylight into a building include the following:

Optimize morning light by designing patient rooms to face east. Studies show that morning light is more effective than evening light in improving patient outcomes.[3]

Include skylights, windows, atriums, and other design elements throughout the building to provide patient and staff access to natural light

Provide adequate artificial lighting in patient care areas and throughout the facility. Staff should have adequate light to clearly see medication labels, charts, computer keyboards, and so forth. This light should be directed so that staff can use it without waking or disturbing patients. Some organizations prefer to use indirect artificial lighting because it still provides the benefits of light while creating a more home-like ambiance.

Move toward a decentralized design. Many health care facilities have a central nurses' station on each unit where charts, orders, medications, and supplies are stored. Nurses in these facilities spend significant time walking up and down hallways to gather what they need for patient care. A recent study by Ann Hendrich and her colleagues used video cameras to track how nurses spend their day. They found, on average, nurses spent only about 30 to 40 minutes of their shifts actually giving care at the bedside because of the time spent searching for and gathering supplies.[11] In addition to pulling nurses away from patient care, crowded, noisy workstations add to staff stress, reduce effective communication, and can lead to medical errors. Decentralized floor plans allow nurses to work closer to patients, thus reducing the need to hunt for supplies. Evidence shows that these floor plans can reduce staff stress, increase satisfaction, and allow nurses to respond more quickly to patient needs.[11]

Evidence-based design incorporates several design principles that have been shown to improve patient safety, patient outcomes, staff performance, and overall satisfaction. Some of the major design principles that make up evidence-based design include the following:

- *Build private rooms*
- *Reduce noise*
- *Incorporate nature*
- *Use wayfinding systems*
- *Improve air quality*
- *Encourage hand washing*
- *Include natural light*
- *Decentralize design*

A Healing Design

Many of the previously mentioned aspects of evidence-based design—daylighting, noise reduction, and access to nature—can work together to provide a healing environment for patients. Other aspects of facility design that promote healing include the following:

Art. Like nature, artwork can reduce patient stress and promote positive feelings. However, the impact of art on the patient is related to the type of art used. Artwork that depicts nature scenes, such as flowers, seascapes, and mountains, can promote positive feelings and reduce stress. On the other hand, abstract art can acutely increase stress and negatively impact patient outcomes.[3]

Music. Soft music can reduce stress and increase positive feelings in a health care environment. Grand pianos playing in lobbies and relaxing music in patient care areas can provide a home-like environment and improve patient well-being.

Social interaction areas. These are places where families and patients can come together, interact, communicate, and support each other. Libraries, kitchens, lounges, activity rooms, gardens, and chapels can all provide places for social interaction.

Home-like designs. Many health care facilities today are cold, impersonal spaces that seem to communicate a lack of caring. By incorporating soft colors on the walls, comfortable furniture, indirect lighting, artwork, and so forth, organizations can communicate that the health care facility is a healing and supportive environment, where staff members care for patients and value their well-being.

Meeting Needs of Staff

The average registered nurse in the United States is more than 43 years old. By 2010, the average age of nurses in this country will increase to 50, and the nurse turnover rate will average 20% each year.[9] The current nursing shortage that plagues the country can be attributed to a variety of factors, including work environments, compensation levels, and the culture of many health care organizations.

As previously mentioned, noisy, stressful, cheerless work environments contribute to staff fatigue, stress, burnout, and poor performance. These environmental factors are pushing up nurse turnover rates. The evidence-based and safety design strategies discussed earlier in this chapter not only can help patients, but can also positively affect staff. For example, a decentralized floor plan, reduced noise, adequate light, and home-like amenities that promote a calm and relaxed environment can improve staff satisfaction, limit fatigue

SIDEBAR 1-3.
The Pebble Project

Launched in 2000, the Pebble Project is a joint research effort between the Center for Health Design and several leading health care providers. Organizations participating in the Pebble Project measure the effect of evidence-based design principles on different quality-of-care and financial performance outcomes. Each participant in the Pebble Project defines particular outcomes to measure, but mostly the outcomes center on areas of clinical improvement, patient and family satisfaction, organizational change, and financial performance. Some measures that organizations use include the following:

- The number of patient falls
- The number of patient transfers
- Infection rates
- The number of medical errors
- The rate of employee turnover
- The use of pain medication

The goal of the Pebble Project is to create a "ripple effect" through health care, so that more organizations investigate and implement evidence-based design principles.[12]

and burnout, enhance performance, and increase staff retention. Respite areas, such as gardens, music rooms, and chapels, can provide a place for staff to rejuvenate and recharge before returning to work.

Following are additional ways that organizations can improve the work environment through design:

Mobile charting. An organization can increase staff efficiency and reduce fatigue by using mobile charting. Mobile charting stations can be moved about a unit and docked at "charting islands." This allows quick access to patient information and flexibility for patient care.[14]

Cushioned flooring materials. Because nurses spend the majority of their day on their feet, the type of flooring material used in a health care facility can impact the comfort, health, and safety of staff. Cushioned materials, such as carpet or sheet vinyl with a padded backing, can dramatically improve the performance and satisfaction of staff.

Ergonomically designed nurses' stations. Shelves that are too high, outlets that are too low, or computer workstations that stress the hands and wrists can all lead to worker injuries, absenteeism, and an unsafe work environment. Organizations that design environments to limit staff reaching, bending, twisting, and stretching can improve staff safety, health, and satisfaction. More information on ergonomic design can be found in Chapter Three.

Adequate space for medication rooms. To prevent errors and increase patient safety, organizations should design medication rooms so that nurses have adequate space to fully enter the room and close the

SIDEBAR 1-4.
Standardizing for Safety

By standardizing patient room layouts, an organization can prevent medical errors because staff members know the exact layout of a patient room, no matter which room they are in. The time spent searching for equipment, supplies, and so forth is thus contained. This also reduces staff fatigue and allows caregivers to more specifically focus their attention on patient care. Other ways to enhance patient and staff safety in design include the following:

Increase patient visibility. By designing rooms so the staff can easily see the patients, an organization can decrease the likelihood of falls.

Encourage automation when possible. By reducing the reliance on human memory, organizations can ensure that tasks are successfully completed on time. This reduces the chance for mistakes that are caused by stress, fatigue, lack of communication, and other human factors.

Address specific types of events. By designing to proactively address potentially problematic events, such as medication errors, patient falls, inpatient suicides, and wrong-site surgeries, organizations can specifically reduce potential hazards that threaten patient safety.

Chapter Three addresses the specifics of a safety-focused design process in greater detail. The work of John Reiling at St. Joseph's Hospital (profiled on pages 50-57) discusses the organization's step-by-step approach to designing for safety.

SIDEBAR 1-5.
Planetree Design

Planetree is a nonprofit organization that advocates for the patient perspective in health care. The Planetree model marries the concept of a healing environment with a patient-centered approach to care. One of the model's nine components focuses on creating a healing environment through design. Planetree encourages health care facilities that use the Planetree model to design layouts that support patient dignity and value human interaction. While these designs incorporate the latest health care technology, the patient is the focus of the design and not the technology. The Planetree model encourages organizations to design uncluttered environments with space for both patients and families. The Planetree model emphasizes the significant impact of social interaction, artwork, and access to nature on patient outcomes.[13]

door. This allows the nurse to prepare medications in a quiet place without distraction.

Similar patient care areas grouped together. Staff spend a lot of time during the day walking between different patient care areas. For example, one patient may need to have an x-ray and a CT scan. If the areas that house these two procedures are not located near each other, a staff member may spend time and energy walking from department to department. Layouts that group together similar patient care areas, such as imaging services, can limit the amount of walking necessary.

Organizations have a responsibility to address staff needs in design, not only because of the safety implications of not addressing staff needs, but also because it is the right thing to do.
Consider the words of one expert: "Think of the impact on the staff of cramped quarters, inadequate lighting and personal storage space, long walks between patient rooms, and distraction-prone work spaces. How can you expect employees to 'go above and beyond' with patients and their families when you haven't provided work environments conducive to the employees' own physical and psychological health?"[16]

SIDEBAR 1-6.
Reducing Absenteeism

In addition to improving staff satisfaction and performance, workplace design can reduce absenteeism. A recent study showed that a healthy indoor climate led to a 2.5% drop in absenteeism across several industries. Although this may seem like a small impact, during the course of a building's 30-year life span, the saved cost from the increase in productivity due to reduced absenteeism can more than match the initial cost of a building's design and construction.[15]

The Business Case for Evidence-Based Design

While the evidence suggests that incorporating design elements, such as access to nature, coordinated wayfinding systems, increased light, artwork, and so forth, can improve patient outcomes and safety, many organizations hesitate to incorporate these design elements because of cost concerns. Some of the previously mentioned suggestions would require capital expenditure; however, the benefits of the suggestions should outweigh the costs. One architect calculates that building a 300-bed hospital with larger, variable-acuity single-patient rooms, decentralized nursing stations, and other elements of evidence-based design would add 5% to the building cost. This may seem like a large expense, but it is estimated that organizations will recoup the cost through decreased patient falls, reduced patient transfers, reduced infections, and limited medical errors.[11] One 56-bed cardiology critical care unit decreased its rate of patient falls by 75% because of a decentralized design. That, coupled with other evidence-based design strategies, is expected to save the organization $17 million a year.[16]

Case Study 1-1, beginning on page 13, illustrates how one organization incorporated evidence-based design strategies into its building project, and the impact these strategies had on the safety and quality of care provided at the organization.

Case Study 1-1. Creating a Healing Environment

Bronson Methodist Hospital's Experience with Evidence-Based Design

For many organizations, building a health care facility from scratch is a dream. New facilities can incorporate state-of-the-art equipment and design strategies and include all the latest technology. In the mid-1990s, Bronson Methodist Hospital, located in Kalamazoo Michigan, was given the opportunity to fulfill its dream. The organization's main facility, built in 1905, was in desperate need of replacement. With a nearly $200 million budget, the organization began a construction project that incorporated a 750,000-square-foot replacement hospital, a medical office building, an ambulatory care pavilion, and a parking ramp for nearly 800 vehicles.

Gathering Information

"We viewed this process as a once-in-a-lifetime opportunity to get the building and culture just right," says Frank Sardone, CEO of Bronson Methodist. "We looked for best practices in literature and conducted our own research to determine the best ways to improve quality and safety in our organization." For example, Bronson conducted several observational studies to determine the work practices and communication patterns of staff. The organization also reviewed both patient and staff satisfaction surveys and conducted focus groups with patients. Bronson Methodist studied many issues and considered a lot of options. "We spent more than five years conducting research, investigating options, and planning," says Sue Reinoehl, vice president of business development for Bronson Methodist.

Choosing the Design Team

Bronson was very particular in choosing its design team. "We wanted to make sure that the architects were able to create the type of environment we were looking for," Sardone says. First the organization reviewed proposals from several different architects and made a list of who would be qualified to do the job. The organization kept winnowing the list until a final list was created. "We actually visited the final list of architects in their offices to ensure they had the culture that would facilitate the type of building process we needed," says Sardone.

To keep the project on track, Bronson created several themes that were kept at the forefront of the project. These themes were often repeated to the project team and staff:

- Create a healing environment
- Ensure ease of access to and within the facility
- Integrate the facility with the surrounding neighborhoods and downtown community

Changing the Culture While Changing the Building

Leadership and staff at Bronson considered the project much more than just building a new facility. "It was an opportunity for profound cultural change, and we seized that opportunity," Sardone says. The organization put the patients' perspective first and shifted the organizational culture to completely focus on the needs, convenience, and safety of patients. Customer service and patient satisfaction took on increased importance throughout the organization. "We used the building as a mechanism for change and implemented several new policies concurrently with the move to the new building," says Reinoehl. For example, to make it easier for patients to distinguish among different types of personnel, Bronson chose new uniforms that were color coded to the staff person's role in the organization. Registered nurses wore one color uniform, while nurses' assistants wore another; technicians wore yet another color, and so forth. This helped patients easily distinguish among different types of staff and improved communication.

Design Strategies

While shifting the culture to a more patient-driven environment, Bronson also designed the physical environment to be patient focused. Design elements included the following:

- Private rooms. All 287 of the organization's inpatient rooms are private. This increases patient and family privacy and satisfaction while decreasing the rate of patient transfers and health care–associated infections.
- Decentralized nursing stations
- The use of light, water, music, and artwork to create a healing environment
- The use of aquariums in waiting rooms, instead of televisions, to cut down on noise and stress

Continued on page 14

Continued from page 13

- Flexibility to incorporate future technologies, such as computerized prescriber order entry

Impact of Design and Cultural Changes

Some critics of evidence-based design feel that changes such as increased light, private rooms, and reduced noise will not have any significant effect on patient outcomes. This has not been the case for Bronson Methodist. The organization conducted a four-year study on the impact of private rooms on health care–associated infection rates. The organization collected data for two years prior to the opening of the new facility and continued to collect data for two years after. The results showed that private patient rooms decreased health care–associated infection rates by 11%. This wasn't the only area impacted by evidence-based design: Patient and staff satisfaction also improved. "We have grown by one third in the past four years and [have] seen high levels of patient, staff, and physician satisfaction. Because of our patient-focused culture, customer service, and design strategies, we are seeing an increased preference, among the public, for our institution," says Sardone. Nursing turnover rates for the organization are now at 4.7%. This is significantly less than the national average of 17%.

Building for the Future

As a result of its growth, Bronson Methodist just approved a $50 million additional development on its campus. The new inpatient pavilion will house obstetrics and some pediatric care units and is scheduled to open in 2007. "We are looking to incorporate the same design strategies in the new building because they are so successful. There is more research now that reinforces the importance of evidence-based design. For example, new research shows that private rooms in the NICU improve patient outcomes," Sardone says.

While most organizations will not get the opportunity to create a $200 million new building, they can incorporate the principles of evidence-based design into their facilities. Evidence-based design can be included in smaller construction or renovation projects, if there is a desire and commitment. Organization leaders must embrace and reinforce the concept of a healing design. In addition, changing the culture of an organization to be more patient driven can further enhance any design strategies incorporated in a new facility.

CASE AT A GLANCE

■ Main challenge

To design a facility that is focused on the needs of patients and can improve quality of care, customer service, and patient satisfaction.

■ Issues

At the time of planning, very few studies addressed the benefits of healing design. Bronson researched best practices and conducted several observational studies to determine the design strategies for the facility.

■ Solutions

Bronson Methodist used several evidence-based design strategies such as private rooms and decentralized nurses' stations to create a healing environment that focused on the needs and perspective of patients. In addition, the organization shifted its culture to be more patient focused and customer-service driven.

■ Outcomes

Because of the use of private rooms, the organization decreased patient transfers and health care–associated infections. This improved patient care and saved the organization money. In addition, the culture and environment worked together to improve market share and enhance patient, staff, and physician satisfaction.

Identifying and Addressing the Needs of the Community

In addition to considering the safety and outcomes of patients and staff, an organization should also consider the health care needs of the community it serves. Demographics, economic influences, and geographic location can all affect the needs of the community and impact the type and design of the construction project.

Changing Demographics

The demographics of communities have changed during the past 50 years. The dynamics of a particular community could be completely different than they were when the community's health care facility was built. For example, steel mills that generated thriving river towns in the 1950s are closing, and many of the people who live in those communities are leaving. The population that could once support a 100-bed tertiary hospital is no longer there.

On the other hand, with the advent of better highway and transportation systems, some areas once considered rural are now being incorporated into suburbs of major metropolitan areas. The population in these "collar counties" is booming, and the small hospital that once adequately served the population is now woefully out of date.

An Aging Population. In addition to the changing dynamics of communities, the national percentage of the population older than 65 is increasing because "baby boomers" are entering retirement. This segment of the population is projected to increase by 100%, from 36 million in 2000 to 72 million in 2030. The population older than 80 is projected to increase by 117% during this time.[17] As the baby boomers age, more of them will need to use health care facilities to treat illnesses. Organizations must prepare for this influx of patients.

A Sicker Population. The patient mix in many health care facilities is also different than it was 50 years ago. Because outpatient facilities can treat more of an individual's basic health care needs, people who do go to a hospital or long term care facility are usually sicker than they were. Newer facilities will need more intensive care units (ICUs) and reduced distances between treatment areas so patients do not need to travel or transfer as often to receive appropriate care. In addition, new diseases such as HIV/AIDS are increasing the need for hospitals to offer the most advanced medical technologies.

A Culturally Diverse Population. While the population is aging, the cultural mixture of communities is also changing. The influence of Hispanic, African American, and Asian cultures on communities has impacted the nature of the health care needed in those communities. For example, different ethnic groups are at greater risk for certain health care conditions, and organizations may need to devote more space to address these conditions. African Americans, for example, are 1.6 times more likely to have diabetes than non-Latino whites.[18] Organizations located in communities with large African–American populations may want to devote more facility space to diabetes care.

In addition to treating certain types of illnesses, organizations with culturally diverse patient populations should consider the impact of different cultures on building design. For example, if English is not the first language for some of its patients, an organization may need to have multilingual wayfinding systems. If the religious diversity of the community warrants, the organization may need to have multiple spaces that address the varying needs of different religions. As the United States becomes more culturally diverse, health care organizations should embrace that diversity and consider it when designing patient care spaces.

TIP

Planning for the Bariatric Patient

The Centers for Disease Control and Prevention (CDC) estimates that 30% of U.S. adults age 20 years and older—more than 60 million people—are obese.[19] An obese patient, also known as a bariatric patient, has several health care facility needs unique to the population. Patient lifts, wider seats in the waiting room, and bigger patient beds are all necessary to effectively treat bariatric patients. When planning a construction project, organizations should keep in mind the needs of bariatric patients and visitors. Despite the efforts of many, Americans are not getting thinner, and the percentage of the population that will need special equipment for basic health care is increasing. ■

Increased Use of the Emergency Department

Changing demographics aren't the only issues affecting community health care needs. The insurance industry affects the health care usage patterns of different communities. As health care costs rise, more and more people are unable to afford health insurance. In 2002 the United States had more than 40 million uninsured individuals, representing 15.2% of the population. In 2003 an additional 1.4 million people lost insurance overage.[17]

One of the effects of this rising uninsured population is the increased use of the emergency department (ED) as a primary source for care. Instead of paying for wellness visits to a primary care physician, more people are waiting until their health demands attention before seeking treatment.

In 2004 there were 125 million emergency room visits, up from 90 million in 1994.[17] People are turning to the ED because the Emergency Medical Treatment and Active Labor Act requires every health care organization providing emergency services to treat a patient, regardless of his or her insurance or payment status. Consequently, individuals who come to the ED can be assured they will receive care regardless of their ability to pay.

Because more people are using the emergency department, many EDs are overcrowded. In some cases patients are being treated in hallways. Organizations should consider how the influx of patients to the ED impacts the design needs of a facility. For example, to accommodate the overflow of patients into the ED, organizations should consider designing facilities with more triage and holding areas. (More discussion on emergency room design and patient surge can be found in Chapter Three.)

The Changing Definition of Need

A need is something that is necessary and required. In the last 50 years, what constitutes a need in this country has changed. Americans are demanding more: better service, more advanced technology, and more extras. What could "wow" someone in 1950 would barely raise an eyebrow today.

With the influence of managed care decreasing, patients have more choices on where to go for their health care needs, and consequently, health care organizations have to compete for market share. To be competitive, some organizations are appealing to the public's need for luxury. Dramatic lobbies, hotel-like surroundings, food-court cafeterias, and upscale coffee shops can all entice patients into a facility, thus improving the organization's bottom line.

What used to be considered a luxury in health care—a private room with space for the family to spend the night—is now expected. In some cases, patients are willing to spend top dollar for private rooms that have all the amenities, such as DVD players, home-like furniture, whirlpool baths, catered food, Internet connections, kitchens, and comfortable spaces for families to stay. These "amenity suites" can drive business to a health care organization, if members of the community can afford such luxury accommodations. The influx of baby boomers who demand such luxuries will require some organizations to consider devoting space to amenity suites.

Alternatives to the Traditional Health Care Facility

Although some health care organizations are designing for luxury, others are facing the significant challenge of providing effective high-quality care with limited resources. Depending on its location, demographics, and economic climate, a community may be forced to close a hospital. This can result in the loss of physicians and other health care personnel in the community. In turn, the loss of skilled health care professionals can limit a community's access to basic primary, urgent, and emergency care services.[20]

To minimize the wholesale closing of small rural health care facilities, the Balanced Budget Act of 1997 authorized the creation of the critical access hospital (CAH) program. This legislation allows for enhanced Medicare reimbursement for facilities located in rural areas that meet certain characteristics (*see* Sidebar 1-7 on this page). By creating the CAH, the government ensured that rural communities could still have easy access to quality health care, without having to produce the capital outlay necessary for a brand new general hospital. For suburban community hospitals that do not qualify for critical access designation, organizations can consider becoming a satellite hospital (*see* Sidebar 1-8 on page 17) to a larger facility.

SIDEBAR 1-7.
Critical Access Hospitals

CAHs are rural hospitals that receive cost-based reimbursement from Medicare. To receive CAH designation, an organization must meet certain criteria:

- Have no more than 25 acute beds
- Have an average annual length of stay of no more than 96 hours
- Be located more than 35 miles from another hospital, within 15 miles from another hospital in mountainous terrain or in areas with only secondary roads, or receive state certification that the facility is a necessary provider of health care services to residents in that area

Should an organization receive CAH designation, it receives 101% of Medicare reimbursement.[21]

Depending on the location and needs of the community, the services provided by a CAH or a satellite hospital may differ. Some of these facilities may include a small inpatient unit, an emergency room with transfer agreements to larger tertiary facilities, diagnostic facilities, and clinical spaces. These facilities can provide opportunities for physicians to telecommute and offer remote diagnostic services. Visiting specialists can have access to office space, exam rooms, and diagnostic equipment. These facilities can also offer community-based support services, such as the following:

- Meeting rooms
- Classrooms
- Exercise rooms
- Medical library
- Diet kitchens

CAHs and satellite hospitals typically do not have to have a pharmacy, administrative offices, or extensive inpatient beds. They can rely on a larger facility with which they contract to provide these services. (*See* Case Study 1-2 beginning on page 18.)

SIDEBAR 1-8.
Satellite Hospital

A satellite hospital may be a remote site of a currently licensed and certified hospital and may operate under the main hospital's certification number. It may be part of a hospital that provides inpatient services in a building also used by another hospital. Or, it may be an entire building of a hospital on the same campus. No matter what its format, a satellite hospital maintains separate admission and discharge records but is serviced by the same fiscal intermediary of the parent hospital. It is treated as a separate cost center of the hospital and maintains separate accounting and statistical data.[21]

To build a CAH or satellite facility is typically less expensive than constructing a small, full-service hospital. While a 30-bed facility may cost $30 million to construct, a CAH with complete ED, diagnostic services, and clinical offices may cost only $5 million.

More than one organization may serve the same population based on geographic location. This may or may not be warranted or sustainable. Instead of fighting over market share, organizations might consider whether two or more health care facilities are necessary for the community, and whether the possibility exists to convert one of the facilities into a more specialized health care center, such as a CAH or satellite hospital.

Organizations choosing to replace an existing facility with one offering more limited services may face some obstacles. Community pride may affect an organization's decision to close down a facility. If a hospital has been in place for 50 years, the community may not want to see it go, even if the care it provides is not as good as a larger, nearby hospital. Organizations will need to present the case to the community that the change is necessary and that moving toward a smaller, more specialized facility can actually serve the community better than a complete rebuild of a larger facility.

SIDEBAR 1-9.
Guidelines for Design and Construction: From Hill-Burton to the American Institute of Architects

One component of the Hill-Burton legislation was a set of guidelines that health care organizations receiving Hill-Burton grants and loans were required to follow during the planning, design, and construction process. In the 1980s, Hill-Burton no longer gave out funds, and the guidelines were removed from the legislation. The American Institute of Architects (AIA) picked up the guidelines, and now a 125-member, interdisciplinary committee updates and revises the guidelines every four years. The Joint Commission references the AIA Guidelines in its "Management of the Environment of Care" (EC) standards; specifically, in EC.8.30, EP 1, as one way of creating sound design.

In addition to discussing the planning, design, and construction of the standard hospital, the guidelines also address the planning, design, and construction of small community hospitals, Critical Acess Hospitals (CAHs), satellite hospitals, and so forth. Individuals can access the guidelines through AIA's Web site, www.aia.org. More information on the AIA guidelines can be found in Chapters Two and Three.

Case Study 1-2. Hospitals Join Forces to Meet the Needs of the Community

In 1993 Barnes Hospital and Jewish Hospital, adjacent urban hospitals affiliated with Washington University School of Medicine in St. Louis, and Christian Health Services, a suburban community hospital network, merged to form BJC HealthCare. The merger resulted in one of the largest nonprofit health care organizations in the United States. One of the goals of the new organization was to create a regional health care system, in which rural communities outside St. Louis could have access to the same level of high-quality health care that was offered in the St. Louis metropolitan area. BJC approached several rural hospitals and asked them to participate in the regional system. Two of these facilities were Bonne Terre Hospital and Farmington Hospital.

Located 12 miles from each other, the two hospitals, along with one other, served the residents of St. Francois County in southeastern Missouri. Farmington Community Medical Center was the larger of the two facilities with 130 beds. It was located in the county seat, which had nearly 14,000 residents. The hospital had an average daily census of 50 patients. Bonne Terre Hospital was located in a small town of fewer than 5,000 people. The hospital had 69 beds, with an average daily census of 20. Despite their convenient locations within the St. Francois community, neither organization reached 20% of the county's population. In fact, many county residents (almost 40%) were choosing not to use Farmington or Bonne Terre Hospital (or the third hospital, Mineral Area Regional Medical Center) and were leaving the county and going elsewhere for their medical needs.

Affiliation with BJC offered the facilities a solution. They would merge to become one hospital with two sites and become part of BJC's regional network. To drive the merger, BJC gave Farmington capital funds to augment its facilities and equipment. With a $19 million capital investment from BJC, Farmington became a state-of-the-art, 70-bed, full-service hospital. BJC also gave capital funds to Bonne Terre, but with different expectations. With a $5 million capital investment, Bonne Terre rebuilt its facility with fewer beds and more limited services. "Bonne Terre is akin to 'hospital lite.' The new facility has a state-of-the-art emergency department and diagnostic services, but it only has three inpatient beds," says John Reeve, president of Christner, Inc., the St. Louis architectural firm in charge of planning and designing both new facilities.

Joining Forces to Deliver Care

In exchange for the capital funds from BJC, Bonne Terre and Farmington became part of the BJC HealthCare network. Now known as Parkland Health Center Bonne Terre and Parkland Health Center Farmington, the two organizations serve the St. Francois community by sharing resources and targeting the needs of the population. Both organizations have an emergency department (ED), diagnostic services, and a primary care facility. In addition, Farmington houses the following services for both organizations:

- Administration
- Pharmacy
- Dietary
- Medical records
- Material services/stores
- Engineering

Although this merger was started before the critical access hospital (CAH) legislation was passed, Bonne Terre did apply and qualify for CAH designation.

Designing for the Community

The design of Bonne Terre addresses the needs of the community, without over-duplicating services. With Farmington Hospital only a short distance away, residents of Bonne Terre do not need a full-service general hospital within their town. However, during an emergency, 12 miles can seem quite long. With a 24-hour/7-days-a-week emergency room, Bonne Terre residents can have ready access to emergency services. Although not designed to fully treat trauma patients, the organization is set up to stabilize and transfer trauma patients to Farmington Hospital or BJC hospitals in St. Louis.

Bonne Terre is designed to be flexible. For example, the three inpatient beds that are located next to the ED can be used as inpatient beds or for overnight observation, if necessary. The community rooms, included in the original design of the facility, were designed to be converted into clinical areas should the need arise. Since the building of Bonne Terre, the community rooms have been

Continued on page 19

Continued from page 18
converted into clinical areas for infusion and a sleep clinic. The building also includes outpatient clinic space. Specialists within the BJC system see patients in this suite on a rotating basis.

To serve the community, Bonne Terre also offers basic diagnostic services, such as x-rays, mammography, basic laboratory services, and so forth, but the facility does not offer low-volume and/or high-cost services, such as surgery, obstetrics and nursery, and advanced imaging. Part of the economic model of the facility was to arrange a plan that made the basic support services conveniently available to the ED while also being supported by daytime volume generated by the outpatient clinic. Should an individual need more advanced diagnostics, he or she is referred to Farmington or on to St. Louis.

Gaining Community Support

"One of the challenges with this process was getting the community on board," Reeve says. "Many people in the Bonne Terre community felt they were losing their hospital and were resistant to change. It took many years to gain community support." BJC brought together people from the Farmington and Bonne Terre communities to discuss their needs. It was clear that St. Francois County did not need both facilities operating as full-service general hospitals. The cost and duplication of efforts would be too great. By creating a more streamlined facility at Bonne Terre, the residents of Bonne Terre could have their basic needs met efficiently, without having to raise funds for a new general hospital. The residents would have access to a brand new facility that could serve their emergency and diagnostic needs, and the transfer agreements with Farmington allowed residents of the community to have access to the most current health care procedures and technology. Through discussions with BJC, it became clear to community leaders that Bonne Terre would not "lose" its hospital, but just readjust its services to better meet the needs of the community.

As a result of BJC's involvement, Bonne Terre Hospital and Farmington Hospital went from two old facilities in desperate need of improvement to one state-of-the-art health care delivery system with two sites. The care provided by the two facilities is more streamlined, convenient, up to date, and efficient. Community residents are satisfied with the arrangement and are assured of receiving the most appropriate and highest-quality care.

CASE AT A GLANCE

■ Main Challenge

To provide efficient and up-to-date care for a rural county.

■ Issues

St. Francois County had two small hospitals in desperate need of renewal and repair. The communities these hospitals served did not have the funds to renovate the hospitals or build new ones. BJC HealthCare, a large health care system in St. Louis, was looking for ways to expand the care it provided into rural communities.

■ Solutions

BJC partnered with Farmington and Bonne Terre Hospitals to create an integrated health care delivery system with two sites. Bonne Terre provides limited services and refers patients to Farmington when necessary. Farmington houses the major support services for the two facilities. Both organizations refer patients to BJC, if warranted.

■ Outcomes

The St. Francois community is adequately served by BJC and the new facilities. Between the three organizations, members of the community receive the same comprehensive, high-quality care as their urban counterparts.

Assessing the Needs of the Community

The previous sections discuss the value of determining a community's needs for health care before planning the type and design of a health care facility. Several ways to assess the needs of a community exist, including the following:

- Examine health care use data, which is typically available from the public health department
- Examine third-party health care use data. Some private companies have databases of health care usage based on insurance claims. For a fee, organizations can obtain data for their community.
- Review census data, available from the U.S. Census Bureau, on the changing demographics of the community
- Conduct community surveys, meetings, or focus groups that assess the community's needs and perceptions of the current health care organization
- Conduct patient and staff surveys, meetings, or focus groups to gather feedback on the performance and services offered by the health care facility

Based on the results of this data, an organization can gain a better understanding of the needs of the community and what type of facility is necessary to meet those needs.

Incorporating Changes in Technology

Tremendous technological advances in health care have occurred in the past 50 years, and the future looks bright for increased technological improvements. The advent of computers, the Internet, imaging technology, and the laser have all significantly affected the practice of medicine.

To remain competitive and ensure the highest quality of care, organizations need to design new buildings, renovation projects, and additions to accommodate current technology. Organizations that do not embrace technology will soon be unable to compete for the consumer's health care dollar. These designs must also be flexible enough to add new technology in the future. Some areas of technology to consider when planning a facility include the following:

Equipment. MRIs, CT scanners, PET scanners, ultrasound machines, and so forth are relatively new technology, and many health care facilities were not built to house this equipment. Organizations will need to create adequate and appropriate spaces for such equipment and allow flexibility as the technology improves and changes.

Computer-based technology. Computers are being used to communicate, store information, and prevent errors in health care. For example, pharmaceutical bar-coding technology, computerized prescriber order entry systems, automated medication dispensing units, and computerized medical records all require computers to function. Even more basic than that, e-mail systems and Internet search functions all require staff to have access to computers. Facility design should allow for centralized computer servers, computer terminals in patient rooms, docking stations for handhelds and laptops, portable charting stations, workstations in physician offices, and so forth. Because technology has become so portable, there is less of a need for a centralized nursing station for patient monitoring and more of a need for areas adjacent to patient rooms for charting and observation.

Coverage. In today's era of wireless communications and networking, the coverage of wireless devices, cellular phones, and computers should be a consideration.

More technically advanced procedures. Medicine and technology are both advancing at phenomenal rates. Consequently, a host of new technologically complex procedures have been created. In addition, many current procedures are becoming more technical. For example, open heart surgery and laser surgery are more common than ever before and yet both procedures are highly technical. Surgery and imaging are merging. Designers will have to work with clinicians to design surgical suites, patient care rooms, and diagnostic areas to accommodate both current and future advances in medicine.

TIP

Bar-Coding Systems Require More Accessible Storage

Many health care organizations are moving toward bar-coded medications. This technology will allow health care organizations to receive "just-in-time" shipments of medications. Because a bar-coded medication is scanned prior to patient administration, the computer system can document how much supply remains and whether a need to order more exists. New supplies are brought into the facility on an as-needed basis. This automated system decreases the need for central storage areas in health care facilities. However, organizations should plan for smaller storage areas on each floor that staff can access quickly to obtain needed supplies. ■

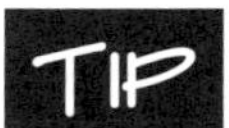

In today's era of cellular phones and wireless networks, it is important that organizations ensure the electromagnetic compatibility of equipment. Telemetry equipment, used to monitor patients' vital signs, is particularly susceptible to electromagnetic interference (EMI). Telemetry monitoring capabilities have expanded so vastly that the potential to receive interference and unintended signals has ballooned. For patients, the consequences of interference with telemetry equipment can be dire. Interference can lead to unreliable monitoring, including potentially missed alarms and even missed life-threatening events. For example, if a patient is being monitored for cardiac arrhythmia and an event occurs, this event may be captured at the patient-worn transmitter, but because of interference, not actually be transmitted to the central monitoring system. In addition, a life-threatening event such as low heart rate may be masked by interference or may not be transmitted to the central monitors.[22]

Organizations can prevent EMI by conducting an assessment of risks associated with new and existing equipment. Organizations must design facilities to minimize interference, choose equipment that limits interference, select an appropriate bandwidth for equipment, and coordinate with local users to prevent interference. ■

The key component in designing for technology is flexibility. Twenty-five years ago, a computer could take up an entire room. Now, you can fit one in the palm of your hand. What will the next 50 years bring? Organizations must be careful to design a facility so that it is not out of date by the time it is built. By designing in flexibility, organizations can be prepared to incorporate new technology as it becomes available. For example, when planning the ED, operating rooms, and ICUs, organizations should ask how these areas could expand to accommodate new technology, if needed. Building these units on outside walls with a clear space for expansion can help the facility remain flexible. Planning for space that can be adapted for other uses later is also beneficial. For example, designing community rooms that can be convert for other uses, should the need arise, can allow the facility to remain flexible. Modular expansions for flexible spaces that are needed quickly, such as ED expansions, are also becoming increasingly popular.

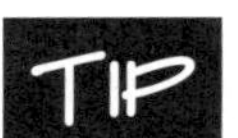

Remember HIPAA

Passed in 1996 to help people buy and keep health insurance even when they have serious health conditions, the Health Insurance Portability and Accountability Act (HIPAA) sets basic requirements that health care organizaitons must meet. A main component of the law addresses patient privacy and confidentiality.

When designing space, organizaitons should keep in mind the privacy requirements dictated by HIPAA. Particularly when designing modular or convertible space, organizations should make sure that the space allows staff to provide care, treatment, and services without infringing upon the patient's privacy. In addition, technology that could house patient information, such as computer terminals or charting stations, should be placed away from public view. Staff, visitors, or other patients should not be able to see patient information when walking by the room.

Because states can and have modified and expanded upon the provisions found in HIPAA, consumer protections vary from state to state. Before beginning design, organizations should examine the HIPAA requirements as they apply to their facility. ■

Environmental Considerations

"First, do no harm" is a tenet of health care as part of the Hippocratic Oath, which all physicians take upon graduation from medical school. It guides the decision-making process of many clinicians regarding patient care. The phrase is also appropriate for the facilities in which clinicians work. Buildings and the building process should not harm patients or the environment, and in fact should do the opposite. In other words, health care facilities should not, under the guise of patient care, pollute the air, leach chemicals into the water, overburden landfills, and so forth. Unfortunately, many health care buildings do not successfully balance patient care with environmental considerations.

In the United States, buildings account for 36% of total energy use, 30% of raw materials use, and 30% of waste output.[23] While these statistics encompass all types of buildings, health care facilities certainly contribute significantly to these numbers. By keeping the environment in mind during the planning and design process, organizations can reduce these numbers and still provide quality health care.

When planning a construction project, organizations should consider how the project and the resulting entity will impact the environment. Threats to the environment can affect not only current patient and staff health and safety, but also the health and safety of future generations.

Sustainable Design

Considering the environment in the design of construction projects is often referred to as "sustainable design." According to the United Nations World Commission on Environment and Development, sustainable design "implies meeting the needs of the present without compromising the ability of future generations to meet their own needs."[24]

The concept of sustainable design has come to the forefront in the last 20 years. It recognizes that human beings are an integral part of the natural world, and nature must be preserved and perpetuated if the human community itself is to survive. Sustainable design requires organizations to think outside the traditional ways and focus on environmental stewardship, social responsibility, and economic viability. The sustainable design approach recognizes the effects of every design choice on the natural and cultural resources of local, regional, and global environments.[25]

Sustainable design requires organizations to consider the impact of design decisions on the environment. It balances the needs of patients with the impact on the environment, so that organizations can adequately meet patient needs while not overtaxing the natural resources of the community.

Historically, the health care industry has been reluctant to pursue sustainable design initiatives. There has been a misperception that sustainable design is not possible in health care. This belief stems from the premise that achieving sustainable outcomes requires compromising patient safety and health. Although certain areas of sustainable design are not appropriate in health care facilities, many sustainable outcomes can be achieved by minor changes in the design process. For example, certain building materials are more hazardous to the environment than others. By choosing more environmentally friendly materials, health care organizations can make a small contribution to preserving the environment. Or, by designing recycling areas in health care buildings, organizations can make recycling possible for the staff, thus eliminating some of the large volume of waste that a health care organization produces.

Depending on the type of project, organizations can incorporate sustainable design principles in a variety of ways during design and construction. Following are a few ways that organizations can use sustainable design principles. This is not an exhaustive list, but one that is meant to provide a starting point for consideration.

- Use recycled/recyclable building materials to divert materials from landfills
- Use local materials in building to eliminate the need to transport materials from significant distances
- Design landscapes to shade buildings and be water efficient. Shade can reduce the amount of air-conditioning needed to cool a building and water-efficient landscapes can reduce the amount of water needed to keep foliage alive.
- Use energy-efficient equipment, such as heating and cooling systems, washers and dryers, and so forth. This reduces the amount of energy consumed by the building.
- Design interiors to use natural lighting. Not only has this been shown to improve patient outcomes and staff morale, but it can reduce the reliance on artificial light and limit light pollution and energy costs.
- Use low-emitting materials to prevent off-gassing of volatile organic compounds (VOCs) and carcinogens into the air. Many building materials emit odors, gases, and toxins. Some of these are relatively harmless and can result, for example, in minor headaches and patient and staff complaints. Others are more critical and can cause serious illnesses, such as cancer. By using low-emitting materials, organizations can limit the amount of dangerous toxins released into the environment, especially into the indoor air, which can be much more polluted than outdoor air and can affect patients (particularly those with weakened immune systems) and staff. In addition to using low-emitting materials, "baking" the new building by elevating the heat to 80° F to 85° F has become a common method of reducing toxins and speeding drying times.
- As previously noted, include recycling centers in convenient locations, thus encouraging patients and staff to recycle. This can reduce the reliance on incineration and thus reduce the amount of airborne dioxin, a potent human carcinogen, released into the air. Incineration also releases mercury, a potent neurotoxin, into the environment.

The Benefits of Building Green

By considering the environment during the planning, design, and construction phases of a project, organizations can reap tremendous benefits. The following are just a few:

Lower energy costs. Reduced energy use is an important economic benefit of sustainable design. Often, organizations can reduce their energy use by improving the building envelope and using more energy-efficient equipment in the building.

Employee recruiting and retention. Because of the current nursing shortage, recruiting quality employees can be a challenge for many health care organizations. The quality of the space in which prospective employees will be working, including such features as daylighting, views to the outdoors, and indoor air quality, can have a significant impact on recruitment efforts. Because green buildings can be more pleasant to work in, organizations might experience less employee turnover, reduced absenteeism, and increased worker productivity.

Improved patient and staff health. Green buildings are healthier buildings. As already noted, the materials used in the building emit fewer hazardous toxins. Pollution is reduced through proper air ventilation and filtration. All these factors make a green building healthier. A healthier building can lead to better patient outcomes and healthier staff.

Tax credits and other incentives. A few states and municipalities offer tax credits and other financial incentives to organizations that build green buildings or reduce their energy use. New York, New Jersey, Maryland, and Oregon are among states that offer significant green building tax credits. Also, a growing number of municipalities offer incentives for green building. In addition, California and several Midwestern states offer energy use rebates.

Positive public image. The positive public image that can result from a commitment to healthy, environmentally responsible facilities can be tremendously beneficial to a health care organization. Coupled with the fact that buildings that include daylighting and cleaner air can actually improve patient outcomes, a green facility can increase market share for a health care organization.[26]

Resources for Sustainable Design Ideas

Before beginning a construction project, organizations should investigate what types of interventions they can use to protect the environment. Some sources of information on sustainable design include the following:

- American Society for Health Care Engineering (ASHE)
- Environmental Protection Association (EPA)
- U.S. Green Building Council (USGBC)
- The Center for Maximum Building Potential
- Hospitals for a Healthy Environment (H2E)

USGBC's LEED Program. One significant voice in the sustainable design movement is the U.S. Green Building Council (USGBC). This nonprofit organization is made up of a coalition of leaders from across the building industry who work to promote buildings that are environmentally responsible, profitable, and healthy.

To help organizations assess how environmentally friendly their building projects are, the USGBC developed the Leadership in Energy and Environmental Design (LEED) program. This program provides a framework for assessing building performance and measuring sustainability goals. It offers third-party certification, professional accreditations, training, and resources. To receive LEED certification, organizations submit an application to the USGBC at the end of their building project. The USGBC assesses the project for compliance with up to 69 points divided into the following six categories:

1. Sustainable Sites
2. Water Efficiency
3. Energy and Atmosphere
4. Materials and Resources
5. Indoor Environmental Quality
6. Innovation and Design Process

To become LEED certified, a facility must receive at least 26 points and meet 7 prerequisites (*see* Figure 1-1 on pages 24-25). Silver certification requires 33 points. The gold and platinum certifications require 39 points and 52 points, respectively. An organization can seek LEED certification for new construction projects, commercial interiors (remodeling projects) or for an existing building. (*See* Case Study 1-3 on pages 26-27 for one organization's journey toward LEED certification.)

FIGURE 1-1. Registered Project Checklist

LEED — LEADERSHIP IN ENERGY & ENVIRONMENTAL DESIGN

Version 2.1 Registered Project Checklist
Project Name:
City, State:

Yes	?	No			
❑	❑	❑	**Sustainable Sites**		**14 Points**
☑	❑	❑	Prereq 1	**Erosion & Sedimentation Control**	Required
❑	❑	❑	Credit 1	**Site Selection**	1
❑	❑	❑	Credit 2	**Urban Redevelopment**	1
❑	❑	❑	Credit 3	**Brownfield Redevelopment**	1
❑	❑	❑	Credit 4.1	**Alternative Transportation, Public Transportation Access**	1
❑	❑	❑	Credit 4.2	**Alternative Transportation, Bicycle Storage & Changing Rooms**	1
❑	❑	❑	Credit 4.3	**Alternative Transportation, Alternative Fuel Vehicles**	1
❑	❑	❑	Credit 4.4	**Alternative Transportation, Parking Capacity and Carpooling**	1
❑	❑	❑	Credit 5.1	**Reduced Site Disturbance, Protect or Restore Open Space**	1
❑	❑	❑	Credit 5.2	**Reduced Site Disturbance, Development Footprint**	1
❑	❑	❑	Credit 6.1	**Stormwater Management, Rate and Quantity**	1
❑	❑	❑	Credit 6.2	**Stormwater Management, Treatment**	1
❑	❑	❑	Credit 7.1	**Landscape & Exterior Design to Reduce Heat Islands, Non-Roof**	1
❑	❑	❑	Credit 7.2	**Landscape & Exterior Design to Reduce Heat Islands, Roof**	1
❑	❑	❑	Credit 8	**Light Pollution Reduction**	1

Yes	?	No			
❑	❑	❑	**Water Efficiency**		**5 Points**
❑	❑	❑	Credit 1.1	**Water Efficient Landscaping, Reduce by 50%**	1
❑	❑	❑	Credit 1.2	**Water Efficient Landscaping, No Potable Use or No Irrigation**	1
❑	❑	❑	Credit 2	**Innovative Wastewater Technologies**	1
❑	❑	❑	Credit 3.1	**Water Use Reduction, 20% Reduction**	1
❑	❑	❑	Credit 3.2	**Water Use Reduction, 30% Reduction**	1

Yes	?	No			
❑	❑	❑	**Energy & Atmosphere**		**17 Points**
☑	❑	❑	Prereq 1	**Fundamental Building Systems Commissioning**	Required
☑	❑	❑	Prereq 2	**Minimum Energy Performance**	Required
☑	❑	❑	Prereq 3	**CFC Reduction in HVAC&R Equipment**	Required
❑	❑	❑	Credit 1	**Optimize Energy Performance**	1 to 10
❑	❑	❑	Credit 2.1	**Renewable Energy, 5%**	1
❑	❑	❑	Credit 2.2	**Renewable Energy, 10%**	1
❑	❑	❑	Credit 2.3	**Renewable Energy, 20%**	1
❑	❑	❑	Credit 3	**Additional Commissioning**	1
❑	❑	❑	Credit 4	**Ozone Depletion**	1
❑	❑	❑	Credit 5	**Measurement & Verification**	1
❑	❑	❑	Credit 6	**Green Power**	1

Yes	?	No			
❑	❑	❑		**Materials & Resources**	**13 Points**
☑	❑	❑	Prereq 1	**Storage & Collection of Recyclables**	Required
❑	❑	❑	Credit 1.1	**Building Reuse, Maintain 75% of Existing Shell**	1

Continued on page 25

FIGURE 1-1. Registered Project Checklist, continued from page 24

Yes	?	No			
❑	❑	❑	Credit 1.2	**Building Reuse, Maintain 100% of Shell**	1
❑	❑	❑	Credit 1.3	**Building Reuse, Maintain 100% Shell & 50% Non-Shell**	1
❑	❑	❑	Credit 2.1	**Construction Waste Management, Divert 50%**	1
❑	❑	❑	Credit 2.2	**Construction Waste Management, Divert 75%**	1
❑	❑	❑	Credit 3.1	**Resource Reuse, Specify 5%**	1
❑	❑	❑	Credit 3.2	**Resource Reuse, Specify 10%**	1
❑	❑	❑	Credit 4.1	**Recycled Content, Specify 5% (post-consumer + 1/2 post-industrial)**	1
❑	❑	❑	Credit 4.2	**Recycled Content, Specify 10% (post-consumer + 1/2 post-industrial)**	1
❑	❑	❑	Credit 5.1	**Local/Regional Materials, 20% Manufactured Locally**	1
❑	❑	❑	Credit 5.2	**Local/Regional Materials, of 20% Above, 50% Harvested Locally**	1
❑	❑	❑	Credit 6	**Rapidly Renewable Materials**	1
❑	❑	❑	Credit 7	**Certified Wood**	1

Yes	?	No			
❑	❑	❑	**Indoor Environmental Quality**		**15 Points**
☑	❑	❑	Prereq 1	**Minimum IAQ Performance**	Required
☑	❑	❑	Prereq 2	**Environmental Tobacco Smoke (ETS) Control**	Required
❑	❑	❑	Credit 1	**Carbon Dioxide (CO_2) Monitoring**	1
❑	❑	❑	Credit 2	**Ventilation Effectiveness**	1
❑	❑	❑	Credit 3.1	**Construction IAQ Management Plan, During Construction**	1
❑	❑	❑	Credit 3.2	**Construction IAQ Management Plan, Before Occupancy**	1
❑	❑	❑	Credit 4.1	**Low-Emitting Materials, Adhesives & Sealants**	1
❑	❑	❑	Credit 4.2	**Low-Emitting Materials, Paints**	1
❑	❑	❑	Credit 4.3	**Low-Emitting Materials, Carpet**	1
❑	❑	❑	Credit 4.4	**Low-Emitting Materials, Composite Wood & Agrifiber**	1
❑	❑	❑	Credit 5	**Indoor Chemical & Pollutant Source Control**	1
❑	❑	❑	Credit 6.1	**Controllability of Systems, Perimeter**	1
❑	❑	❑	Credit 6.2	**Controllability of Systems, Non-Perimeter**	1
❑	❑	❑	Credit 7.1	**Thermal Comfort, Comply with ASHRAE 55-1992**	1
❑	❑	❑	Credit 7.2	**Thermal Comfort, Permanent Monitoring System**	1
❑	❑	❑	Credit 8.1	**Daylight & Views, Daylight 75% of Spaces**	1
❑	❑	❑	Credit 8.2	**Daylight & Views, Views for 90% of Spaces**	1

Yes	?	No			
❑	❑	❑	**Innovation & Design Process**		**5 Points**
❑	❑	❑	Credit 1.1	**Innovation in Design: Provide Specific Title**	1
❑	❑	❑	Credit 1.2	**Innovation in Design: Provide Specific Title**	1
❑	❑	❑	Credit 1.3	**Innovation in Design: Provide Specific Title**	1
❑	❑	❑	Credit 1.4	**Innovation in Design: Provide Specific Title**	1
❑	❑	❑	Credit 2	**LEED™ Accredited Professional**	1

Project Totals (pre-certification estimates)	**69 Points**

Certified 26–32 points **Silver** 33–38 points **Gold** 39–51 points **Platinum** 52–69 points

To become LEED certified, a facility must meet 7 prerequisites and get at least 26 points.

Source: U.S. Green Building Council.

Case Study 1-3. Creating a Green Building

One Organization's Pursuit of LEED Certification

In 2000 Boulder Community Hospital (BCH) began planning a construction project to build a new health care facility. Located in Boulder, Colorado, the new facility consists of a hospital and an outpatient services building, which houses mainly physician practices. The hospital has three floors with 60 patient beds. It has a 24-hour emergency department and an intensive care unit and offers surgery, radiology, inpatient pharmacy, and laboratory services. Maternity care and pediatrics are major components of the new campus.

A Desire to Be Sustainable

During the planning stages, BCH investigated pursuing a sustainable design for the project. "An environmental focus is part of the community's culture here in Boulder," says Kristi Ennis, senior associate for Boulder Associates, the firm in charge of medical architecture for the project. "There were people on the hospital's board of directors who were familiar with sustainable design and recognized that's what the community would want."

The organization searched for a design and construction team that would incorporate sustainable design strategies into the planning, design, and construction process. After BCH selected the team, the group came together to discuss how they would incorporate sustainable design into the building process. At first, the team turned to the U.S. Green Building Council for ideas. "We weren't initially pursuing certification; we were looking at the LEED program for ideas and benchmarks to strive for in the design, planning, and construction process. As we got further into the project, we realized that we could attempt certification," Ennis says.

After the organization decided to pursue certification, members of the organization and the design and construction team determined what LEED points would be attempted. The LEED program has several prerequisites without which an organization cannot get certified. For example, organizations must accommodate recycling within the building and must hire a commissioning agent for the commissioning process. BCH's first step was to ensure that it met all the prerequisites.

The organization then identified the points it was going to attempt and set goals to achieve those points. "It is unrealistic to pursue all the points in LEED. Some of them conflict, some are costly, and some of them are not relevant to health care. We needed to determine where to focus our efforts," says Ennis. "It's important to note that sometimes points attempted will not be achieved. For example, an organization may strive to increase the amount of construction waste that is diverted from a landfill, and a project team can make every effort to achieve this point, but until the project is over, the exact amount of waste diverted will be unknown. The only way to really know if you will earn the point is after the fact, and by then it's too late to change anything. Therefore, it is necessary to commit to attempting a few more points than the team desires, so as to earn the necessary points for certification at the completion of the project."

Focusing Efforts

As previously mentioned, LEED certification is broken down into six categories, within which organizations can pursue different points. The categories are as follows:

- Sustainable Sites
- Water Efficiency
- Energy and Atmosphere
- Materials and Resources
- Indoor Environmental Quality
- Innovation and Design Process

While BCH pursued points in all these categories, the organization focused its efforts on the Energy and Atmosphere, Materials and Resources, and Indoor Environmental Quality categories. "We felt these areas showed the most parallel to a health care organization's primary goals," Ennis says. "Reducing waste and energy use and improving air quality were all areas that health care organizations value." BCH received points in these areas by taking the following actions:

Energy and Atmosphere. The organization built a central utility plant, which housed all the major utility equipment for the facility in one location. Because of the centralization of mechanical equipment, the organization was able to purchase more

Continued on page 27

Continued from page 26

energy-efficient equipment. By housing the equipment in one location, the equipment could run efficiently at all load levels. The additional cost of the central utility plant over a decentralized system was $1.3 million; but with the energy savings accrued from the plant, the organization is projected to recoup the cost in 12 years.

Materials and Resources. BCH supported the local economy during the building process by using local manufacturers and local materials, such as brick, sandstone, and concrete. "In addition to limiting long-distance transportation, the local materials helped the facility fit well into the local vernacular. The exterior design and materials match other buildings in the area," says Ennis. In addition to using local materials, BCH used building materials with recycled content, and the contractor diverted 64% of the construction waste from landfills to recycling facilities.

Indoor Environmental Quality. BCH used building materials with low volatile organic compound (VOC) content. As previously mentioned, VOCs can leech into the environment, and many of them are not healthy; some contain carcinogens. By using low-emitting materials, fewer toxins were released into the indoor environment during construction, and fewer are released during the first few years of building use.

BCH also earned points for their precautionary measures used during construction. "We put cellophane over ducts that were not being worked on to prevent dust from entering them. We also worked to ensure that certain building materials did not get wet, and if they did, then we did not use them in construction," Ennis says.

Submitting for Certification

After Boulder Community Hospital finished its new facility, it submitted its application for LEED certification. Four months after opening, it became the first hospital in the country to receive LEED certification. The facility received 33 points, which garnered silver certification. "While it was a great public relations boost for the hospital, leadership's motivation for seeking certification was to overcome speculation that a health care facility could not be built 'green,'" says Ennis. "The organization wanted to serve as an example of what can be accomplished in health care regarding sustainable design, and the organization leadership hopes that others will realize the possibilities and follow in their footsteps."

The Benefits of LEED

Although LEED certification was appropriate for Boulder Community Hospital, it may not be for other organizations. Even if an organization does not pursue LEED certification, there are definite benefits to examining the LEED checklist (*see* Figure 1-1 on pages 24-25) and incorporating its suggestions into the design process. The checklist can bring up points for discussion and reveal opportunities regarding sustainable design that the organization has not yet considered.

CASE AT A GLANCE

■ Main challenge
To design a facility based on sustainable design principles.

■ Issues
Historically, organizations and design teams have shied away from sustainable design, saying it is not possible in health care. Boulder Community Hospital wanted to serve as an example of how a hospital could consider the environment in planning, design, and construction.

■ Solutions
The organization hired an environmentally focused design team and reviewed the LEED certification checklist for ideas on how to incorporate sustainable design principles into the project. The organization decided to pursue certification and chose a few areas in which to focus its efforts.

■ Outcomes
After the building was completed, Boulder Community Hospital submitted its application for LEED certification. It became the first hospital to receive LEED certification and met its goal of building an environmentally friendly facility.

The Green Guide to Health Care. While the LEED program is useful in assessing how green a building project is, the program was not designed specifically for health care organizations. In March 2003, a professionally and geographically diverse group of green health care industry leaders convened as an independent steering committee to guide development of a "green" certification program for health care. "The ideas in LEED were great, we just needed to make it more applicable to health care," says Robin Guenther, president of Guenther 5 Architects, a member of the steering committee.

The steering committee included representatives from ASHE, The Center for Maximum Potential Building Systems, H2E, and several architecture firms. From this steering group, the *Green Guide for Health Care* was born. The *Green Guide for Health Care* provides health care organizations with a voluntary, self-certifying metric toolkit of best practices that designers, contractors, and organization leadership can use to guide and evaluate their progress regarding sustainable design.[27]

To create the *Green Guide for Health Care,* the steering committee divided into working groups that created each section of the document. Drafted credit language was reviewed and approved by the steering committee as a whole.[27] After a public comment period in which more than 1,200 comments were received, the Green Guide for Health Care began pilot testing in November 2004.

The organizational structure of the *Green Guide for Health Care* was borrowed by agreement from the USGBC's LEED program. With 96 different points and 11 prerequisites (as opposed to LEED's 69 points and 7 prerequisites), the *Green Guide for Health Care* highlights the most relevant environmental issues for health care organizations to consider during planning, design, and construction. For many credits, the *Green Guide for Health Care* directly incorporates the language of the parallel LEED credit. In some cases, existing LEED credits have been modified to respond to the unique needs and concerns of health care facilities. In others, new credits have been added beyond those in current LEED products.[27] For example, because hospitals use a great deal of energy, providing 5% of that energy via on-site renewable energy such as photo voltaics would be fairly costly and large. The *Green Guide to Health Care* revises this requirement to give credits for 1% and 2% renewable energy, thus encouraging smaller efforts.

While the *Green Guide for Health Care* is an evolving process, organizations, at the very least, can use it as a point of discussion about sustainable design issues. The time to think about these issues is before the design phase begins. The type of design team an organization chooses is predicated on its desire to incorporate sustainable design ideas into the overall building process. A complete and current version of the *Green Guide for Health Care* can be found at http://www.gghc.org.

Conclusion

Building a health care facility is a tall order and one that should not be taken lightly. This chapter has introduced myriad considerations that organizations should keep in mind when planning a construction project. To effectively include these considerations in the design and construction process, organizations must have support and buy-in from leadership, including CEOs, boards of directors, and so forth. Without leadership support, the best intentions will remain just intentions. Likewise, input and support from clinical staff, patients, and the community is also valuable. Bringing leadership, clinicians, nonclinical staff, community leaders, architects, and contractors together to discuss considerations before beginning the building process can ensure that the final product incorporates the features that are needed and desired by the organization and its constituents.

The considerations discussed in this chapter are admittedly "blue sky," yet to be on the cutting edge of health care design and remain viable well into the twenty-first century, organizations have an obligation to examine the possibilities of including evidence-based, patient-focused, safety-driven, and sustainable design principles in design and construction. Many organizations are successfully incorporating these principles into their current design schemes. The decisions an organization makes today regarding its facility will have long-term effects, as the health care facilities built today will impact generations to come.

REFERENCES

1. Flower J.: The evidence on evidence-based design. *H&HN,* Jan. 1, 2005. http://www.hospitalconnect.com/hhnmag/jsp/articledisplay.jsp?dcrpath=HHNMAG/PubsNewsArticle/data/050125HHN_Online_Flower&domain=HHNMAG (accessed Apr. 20, 2005).

2. Sandrick K.: Clearing the air: Stopping infection through better IAQ control. *Health Facil Manage* May 2001.

3. Ulrich R., et al.: *The Role of the Physical Environment in the Hospital of the 21st Century: A Once-in-a-Lifetime Opportunity.* A Report to the Center for Health Design and the Robert Wood Johnson Foundation, Sep. 2004. http://www.healthdesign.org/research/reports/physical_environ.php (accessed Apr. 25, 2005).

4. Spannaus N.: Ban the HMOs! The principles of the Hill-Burton approach. *American Almanac and The New Federalist,* Jan. 2000. http://members.tripod.com/american_almanac/hillburt.htm (accessed Apr. 20, 2005).

5. Health Resources and Services Administration, U.S. Department of Health and Human Services: *The Hill-Burton Free Care Program.* http://www.hrsa.gov/osp/dfcr/about/aboutdiv.htm (accessed Apr. 21, 2005).

6. Sadler B.: No opportunity wasted: The case for building better hospitals is stronger than ever. *Interiors and Sources Magazine,* Jan./Feb. 2005. http://www.isdesignet.com/Magazine/2005/janfeb/healthdesign_opportunity.html (accessed Apr. 20, 2005).

7. Voelker R.: "Pebbles" cast ripples in health care design. *JAMA* 250:1701–1702, Oct. 2001.

8. Center for Health Design: *Fact Sheet.* http://www.healthdesign.org/aboutus/press/factsheets/ (accessed May 20, 2005).

9. Center for Health Design: Center for Health Design releases findings on how design can improve the standard of care in health care facilities. *AIArchitect,* Feb. 21, 2005. http://www.aia.org/aiarchitect/thisweek05/tw0218/0218bp_pebble.htm (accessed Apr. 20, 2005).

10. Mazer S.: Stop: Reduce errors by creating a quieter hospital environment. *Patient Safety & Quality Healthcare* pp. 36–39, Mar./Apr. 2005.

11. McCarthy M: Healthy design. *Lancet* 364:405–406, Jul. 31, 2004.

12. The Center for Health Design: *What is the Pebble Project?* www.heathdesign.org (accessed Apr. 20, 2005).

13. Gilpin L.: Twenty-five years of Planetree Design. *Healthcare Design* pp. 13–15, Sep. 2003.

14. Leighty J.: Healing by design. *NurseWeek,* Apr. 23, 2003. http://www.nurseweek.com/news/features/03-04/unitfuture.asp (accessed Apr. 20, 2005).

15. Hobstetter D.: In the Fray: Seeing the light about daylight. *Wall Street Journal,* Oct. 19, 2004.

16. Center for Health Design. Design for success: Efficiency and effectiveness through facility design. *Healthcare Financial Management* pp. DE1–DE13, Nov. 2003.

17. Gormley T.C.: Healthcare construction overview. Paper presented at the ASHE conference, Chicago, Mar. 9, 2005.

18. American Diabetes Association: *Diabetes Statistics for African Americans.* http://www.diabetes.org/diabetes-statistics/african-americans.jsp (accessed Apr. 28, 2005).

19. Centers for Disease Control and Prevention: *Overweight and Obesity: Frequently Asked Questions (FAQs).* http://www.cdc.gov/nccdphp/dnpa/obesity/faq.htm#adults (accessed May 1, 2005).

20. Missouri Hospital Association: *Critical Access Hospitals in Missouri.* http://web.mhanet.com/asp/About_MHA/directories/cah_hospitals.asp (accessed Apr. 28, 2005).

21. Unanue E.: Serving the underserved: New design guidelines for small primary inpatient care facilities. Paper presented at the ASHE Conference, Chicago, Mar. 9, 2005.

22. Joint Commission Resources: Risk assessment for medical telemetry interference: December 1, 2005, ends FCC freeze on most popular medical telemetry spectrum. *Environment of Care News,* Oct. 2005.

23. U.S. Green Building Council: *Why Build Green?* www.usgbc.org (accessed May 2, 2005).

24. United Nations General Assembly: *Report of the World Commission on Environment and Development.* 96th plenary meeting, Dec. 11, 1987. http://www.un.org/documents/ga/res/42/ares42-187.htm. (accessed May 2, 2005).

25. National Park Service, U.S. Department of the Interior: *The Principles of Sustainable Design.* http://www.nps.gov/dsc/dsgncnstr/gpsd/toc.html (accessed May 2, 2005).

26. Wilson A.: Making the case for green building. *Environmental Building News* 14, Apr. 2005. http://www.buildinggreen.com/auth/article.cfm?fileName=140401a.xml (accessed May 2, 2005).

27. *Green Guide for Health Care:* About the Green Guide for Health Care. http://www.gghc.org/about.cfm (accessed Apr. 30, 2005).

CHAPTER TWO:

Master Planning and Predesign

THE PREVIOUS CHAPTER DISCUSSES several considerations organizations should keep in mind when planning a construction project, but these considerations are only the first step in the planning process. Organizations must take these considerations, decide which ones, if any, to follow, create a project team, set a budget, and develop an implementation plan. Such a plan should consider a variety of issues, such as functional requirements, safety, space allocation, equipment needs, and schedule. During this planning process, organizations must keep in mind how a construction project will fit into the strategic plan of the organization, as well as its current physical, organizational, social, political, and economic context.

The planning phase involves two types of planning: master planning and predesign.* Master planning involves outlining the goals, strategies, and actions that will carry a facility long into its future. It is a conceptual process that determines the building needs and plans for an organization over time.

Predesign involves planning for a specific building project. Depending on the size of the maximum build out of the site and scope of the project, organizations may engage in both types of planning separately or combine them into one planning process. For example, large hospitals may create a master plan to map out several building projects, each of which will have its own predesign phase. Each of these predesign efforts will be integrated with the master plan to ensure that strategic objectives outlined in the master plan are met. On the other hand, small organizations that are adding a wing to an existing building may engage in master planning and predesign at the same time. This chapter will examine master planning and predesign together, as they share many common elements.

Master planning and predesign are like preparing for a long trip. You need to know why you are traveling, how you are going, who will accompany you, and who you will meet at each key stopping point. You need contingency plans, time, and money. The planning process should involve distinct tasks, benchmarks, and checkpoints to achieve a thoroughly investigated plan that is on time and within budget. Planning should be an interactive process with workshops, meetings, research, and "homework" periods for all participants. Each step in the process should eliminate certain options and, ideally, bring the team closer to agreement on the best alternatives.

The following paragraphs offer several components of the planning process. The scope and nature of the building project will determine whether organizations engage in all these activities, or just some.

SIDEBAR 2-1.
Financial Planning for the Project

The need to plan a facility's financial structure is as important as the plans for its design and construction. Careful financial and data analysis is an integral part of any planning phase. Just as a building's design evolves through the planning and design process, a financial plan for the project must also evolve to reflect the variations of scope and design.

Conduct a Needs Analysis

As a first step in the planning process, organizations may wish to conduct a needs analysis. This will drive decisions during the planning process and help estimate the capital requirements of the project. A thorough needs analysis should involve a detailed assessment for each department or service. For example, as part of a needs assessment for a maternity unit, an organization should examine population projections of women ages 15 to 44, including historical and projected fertility rates by geographic area. Similarly, in assessing the needs of the surgical service, the organization should examine the impact of managed care and estimate what the population-based surgical procedure rate will be in the future.

As part of a needs analysis, an organization should consider conducting marketing studies and demographic analyses. These types of research can help the organization get information on a variety of topics, including the following:

- Service areas
- The payor mix of constituents
- Community perceptions of the facility and a potential construction project
- Appropriate location of a new facility
- Potential lost revenue due to a construction project or relocation of a facility
- The presence and impact of competition

Results from this research should be considered when determining whether to do a construction project, as well as when determining the location, nature, timing, and financial impact of the project.

* Some organizations may call this process Role and Program.

Although it is impossible to anticipate every need and the costs associated with meeting each need, organizations can create a rough estimation to determine organizational priorities. Organizations should consider reexamining their needs analysis regularly as master planning and subsequent predesign and design activities move forward.

An important aspect of planning is programming. *Programming involves determining how the current space of an organization will be adapted or how new space will be designed to meet the needs of the organization. To ensure effective programming, the design team and organization representatives must work together to determine organization needs and the best ways to meet those needs.*

Select the Team

A critical step in the planning process is selecting the project team. This is the group of people who influence and are involved in the planning, design, and construction phases of the project. Every project team consists of two distinct groups: representatives of the organization and the consultants who work on the project. To have a successful planning process, organizations should be aware of the needs, goals, and perspectives of these two groups.

Organization Representatives

On any project team, the organization should be represented by a multidisciplinary group from various areas of the organization. This group should provide information to project consultants and react to a wide variety of proposals made by the consultants. Conversely, the project consultants should work with organization representatives to tailor design and layout ideas to fit the organization's culture and unique nature.

Following are some areas of an organization that may be included on a project team:

Crucial members

- CEO or representative of the executive administration
- Physicians and other practitioners
- Nursing staff
- Infection control staff
- Facilities planning and/or engineering staff
- Established planning or building committees within the institution
- Finance department staff

Members who provide additional input

- Allied health staff
- Pharmacy staff
- Laboratory staff
- Support services staff
- A representative of the board of directors

Members who serve in an advisory capacity

- A representative from the community, such as a patient or family representative or community leader

It is important to include representatives of the departments that will be most directly affected by the construction or remodeling projects because they will have to work in the new or remodeled facility. For organizations that are building something totally new and do not yet have staff for the building, project team members should include the CEO, experts in infection control, facilities management, facility planning, finance, and applicable clinical disciplines.

At its best, the planning process allows staff to feel a sense of ownership in the building effort. The benefits of involving staff in planning frequently include more innovative and appropriate results, as well as greater staff buy-in to and satisfaction with the project.

For the planning process to work all participating staff and consultants must have a common level of understanding. This includes mutually understood goals, some common base of knowledge, shared experiences, and easy communication. Shared literature, research, and field trips to innovative facilities can establish this common ground.

Choosing a Leader. Empowerment of a leader from the organization's representatives is critical to ensure that the planning process moves forward vigorously, on time, and on budget. The team leader must be established as the primary contact and conduit for decisions and the exchange of information. The team leader must be a good manager of people, schedules, changes, surprises, and problems. This person must understand the institution's leaders and their interests or concerns, as well as those of the project team, to know when and how to bring about timely decisions. This person must have the authority, responsibility, and respect of management and the board to make the planning process work.

The Professional Consultants

The other members of the project team are the paid professionals who design and execute the planning, design, and construction phases. The exact makeup of the consultant team will vary according to the scope of the effort, the size of the organization, and the nature of services needed to develop and implement a sound plan. The following list identifies a range of consultants that organizations should consider:

- Architects, including the principal, planner, designer, and program manager
- Engineers, including mechanical, civil, structural, electrical, and plumbing engineers
- Contractors, including the project manager, estimators, and schedulers
- Health care management consultants
- Developers or development consultants
- Financial consultants
- Cost estimators
- Equipment and technology planners
- Specialized consultants, including those specializing in kitchens, furniture, information technology, and security
- Landscape architects
- Interior designers

Choosing the Right Consultants. After establishing what outside professional services are needed, criteria should be developed for selecting the best firms and people for each specialty. One way to do this is to send a Request for Qualifications (RFQ) to a number of qualified firms. The submissions from the RFQ should be reviewed and the 5 to 10 most qualified firms should be invited to submit a Request for Proposal (RFP). The firms submitting RFPs should be invited to participate in an interview process with a selection committee. It is important to make sure that deadlines for submission are set allowing adequate time for firms to respond and prepare for RFQs, RFPs, and interviews. It is important to note that the health care organization does not have to issue a separate RFP for each professional consultant required for the project. Many consultants will create a proposal as a team. For example, architects, engineers, and specialized consultants may make one proposal as a group.

During the interview process, organizations should keep in mind the following criteria:

- *Commitment.* The firm and its principals should be able to demonstrate commitment, interest, and understanding of the client's professional service needs.
- *Location and availability.* The location of the firm, with respect to the site and/or client, and its availability when needed, are important, particularly if the firm will be involved through the construction of a building project. This will make it easier to conduct master planning or other predesign services on a more predictable schedule. After construction begins, it becomes very important for the project leader from the firm to be available on short notice. In some cases, the expertise of local firms is not appropriate for the project. In these cases, a more geographically distant firm with appropriate expertise can team up with a local firm to manage on-site issues.
- *Skill and experience.* The relevant skills, experience, and professional training of the people assigned to the effort are essential. It is important to distinguish between the capabilities of the firm and those of the specific staff who will be assigned. In addition, organizations choosing to pursue certain types of design, such as sustainable, evidence-based, or safety-related design, should choose consultants who are well versed in these areas.
- *Track record.* Prospective firms should be able to demonstrate professionalism, dependability, and a proven record of delivering on time and within budget for comparable clients and types of service.
- *Creativity, ingenuity, and imagination.* The proposed consultant team needs to have demonstrated a high level of these attributes in solving complex problems of a similar nature.
- *Firm size.* The size of the firm should match the size and scope of the work. Small firms can be overwhelmed when the scope of work is too large; large firms carry higher overhead costs that can be difficult to absorb when the scope of services is small.
- *Fee.* The fee structure and rates of compensation are a significant factor in selecting consultants.
- *Culture.* A positive relationship should exist between organizational cultures and the key personnel involved in the effort. For architects and engineers, it can also be important that they have a positive working relationship with each other and have worked together before.

Frequently, the best firms for consideration are found by identifying those that have worked with administrative colleagues of comparable organizations. Occasionally, this informal research will uncover negative experiences. It is important to consider that problems in a consultant/client relationship may be due to client-created situations as often as they are due to consultant-created situations.

Choosing a Leader. It is recommended that professional consultants with significant health facility planning and architectural expertise be engaged to conduct and coordinate the planning process. The planning, programming, and design of health care facilities require a broad perspective and knowledge base. This insight should include an understanding of health care delivery systems and services; an understanding of the impact of planning and design on these services; and an understanding of the build-

SIDEBAR 2-2.
Decision Making

For the project team to operate effectively, a clear chain of command should be established early on. Lack of a structured decision-making process is a major cause of delays. Such delays create situations in which outside consultants, such as architects and engineers, exceed both schedule and fee projections. Organizations may want to include a facilitator on the project team to assist with communication and ensure streamlined decision making.

SIDEBAR 2-3.
Selecting the Contractor

It is important to integrate the contractor or construction manager with the project team at the right point of the planning process. Enlisting the contractor's expertise and suggestions early may prevent costly redesign later. The value of having contractors on board during planning efforts includes having advice on project scheduling and an opinion on construction cost. Contractors can also provide advice on the selection of building systems and constructability issues.

ing and design process. These professionals must be able to take into account the values of the broad range of constituents involved in the process and communicate effectively with each of these groups.

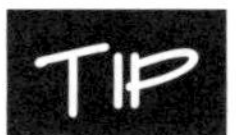

On a fast-moving project, all team members must be able to communicate with each other quickly and effectively. Technology can streamline and enhance communication. For example, interactive sketch pads or drawings can be viewed simultaneously on two or more computers in remote locations. Computer-assisted design (CAD) allows planners and architects to share and easily modify images. CAD drawings of existing facilities should be available during predesign to facilitate analysis of existing space. This is also useful for testing possible solutions to projected needs. A building plan in the form of a CAD document can be modified quickly to evaluate different ideas. ■

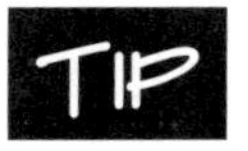

Although organizations can structure the project team in several ways, one way that can be helpful for large construction projects that require input from multiple sources is to use a steering committee and multiple task forces. This method, sometimes called the task force approach, uses a 5-to-10-member steering committee and similarly sized task forces, which focus on specific services or organizational needs. Task forces are organized around specific services (surgery, obstetrics, emergency) and systems (transportation, information, materials). The steering committee includes key decision makers, the architect, the facility planner, medical staff, and possibly members of the board. The committee is responsible for establishing the overall vision and setting budget and scope mandates for each task force. It also resolves conflicting expectations and negotiates trade-offs.

The goal of this approach is to maintain the efficiency and creative potential of a small decision-making team while formalizing the input and participation of departments during the planning of their areas. A disadvantage of splitting project planning participants into separate task force groups is that opportunities for innovative solutions that cut across departmental boundaries may be hindered. This can be minimized by having certain task force members participate in work sessions of other task forces. Another solution is the establishment of a task force with representation from key departments or services that are interdisciplinary in nature. In the absence of these mechanisms, interdisciplinary coordination becomes a role of the steering committee. ■

Collaboration Is the Key. The best projects involve team relationships, shared successes, shared failures, and tolerance for human error and project complexities. Relationships that are adversarial or autocratic are often doomed to failure. Success is much more likely when client and consultants work closely as a team, generating ideas, exploring solutions, discarding bad ideas, and mutually reaching conclusions.

- Planning should always be collaborative. Such collaboration has many advantages, including the following:

- Market, infrastructure, and operation issues are defined early
- Various expertise informs and identifies issues and solutions
- Approval processes are streamlined on every level
- A fact-based case can be made for capital investment[1]

In large projects with many constituencies and finite resources, it is inevitable that conflicting needs will surface during the planning process. Frequent causes of conflict include the relative importance of specific project elements, current needs versus anticipated patient demands, and organizational concepts of the project. The factors forcing these issues are the initial determination of a project budget, sequencing of construction, and the proposed physical location of services. The needs of the surgery service, for example, should be balanced against the needs of other services, including those necessary to support surgery. If these issues are not addressed during this phase, they will reemerge during design, jeopardizing the project scope and timetable, as well as the entire team's morale.

Before beginning the planning process, team members should acquaint themselves with the organization's mission, strategic plan, planning assumptions, and objectives, so there are clear-cut agreements and a mutual understanding of the goals and objectives of planning efforts. This is a good place to begin identifying the organization's existing operational and facility infrastructure.

SIDEBAR 2-4.
Identify Unspoken Goals

When teams begin the planning process, every effort must be made to put all goals on the table. Unstated goals can throw a process off track and result in miscommunication and misunderstandings For example, an organization may have an unstated goal of constructing a building that does not look too expensive, so patients don't raise questions regarding the cost of health care. At the same time, the architect may aspire to win a design award and may focus on design elegance. These unspoken goals need to be candidly shared before a line is put to paper. A shared understanding of building image between architect and client can be achieved by jointly touring notable works of architecture or carefully studying slide images to determine client and community desires.

Collect Data

The data collection process familiarizes the project team with the organization, its services, and its facilities. The process should identify a wide range of goals, facts, and issues that will affect or be affected by the planning, design, and construction process. Data collection activities usually involve detailed graphic and written documentation of the following:

- Existing services
- Operational structures
- Property boundaries and features
- Facilities

Gather Facility-Specific Information

Documenting the layout, size, and function of existing facilities is necessary to understand their current use and condition, as well as the future needs of the facility. As part of this effort, the project team may want to develop narrative and graphic histories of each facility, including changes in the physical plant. The team should look at existing drawings and verify that they are accurate. In some cases, an on-site survey, with measurements of each department, floor, building, and site, may be necessary.

Organizations should evaluate the current physical condition of all existing facilities and review their potential for continued use, whether in their existing form or as renovated space. Three specific areas should be evaluated:

1. *Building systems and infrastructure.* Evaluating the condition of a building involves identifying, or verifying, the types of materials and systems used in the original construction and subsequent renovations of the building, as well as its general condition. Special features or qualities, and notable deficiencies, should be documented. At this point, it may be appropriate to have engineering consultants evaluate the condition, life expectancy, and future capacity of existing buildings, sites, and, perhaps, off-site systems.
2. *Facility compliance with standards and codes.* A code analysis should also be conducted to verify each building's code classification, its allowable occupancy load, its allowable height and area limitations, and its conformance to codes and

SIDEBAR 2-5.
A Change in Direction

The data collection process will undoubtedly reveal new information about the facility and its needs. As knowledge evolves, prior assumptions and concepts may need to be revisited. The need to reconsider early proposals should not be viewed as stepping backward, a failure of the process, or poor planning. An organization or team must never be afraid to pull the plug and reassess the information or process, particularly in this era of rapid change. New ingredients can bring about a different answer. The project team must be willing to change its direction, reassess its assumptions and objectives, or stop the process for design or redesign. It is better to take risks in planning than to build the wrong facility in the wrong place.

standards related to seismic design, life safety, accessibility, and so forth. The results of this assessment often will play a significant role in determining the future use of facilities and their need for renovation or replacement.

3. *The ability of existing facilities to accommodate functional and operational space needs.* Called a functional assessment, this should be made to determine how existing facilities accommodate the functional space needs of each department or service. The process usually involves evaluating surveys conducted during meetings with departmental staff or their representatives on the project team. Information should be gleaned about the services provided by each department and the department's functional relationship with other departments. The functional analysis should consider the location of each department, how accessible each department is, and how location affects the functionality of each department. The bottom line is the functional assessment should analyze whether current departmental space accommodates existing and future needs.

Conduct a Workload Analysis

As part of the data collection process, a project team should conduct a workload analysis. This can project the space needed for specific components of the project, such as operating rooms, patient beds, or examination rooms. If the project scope and size allow, team members may wish to create a five-year profile that details historical workload, staffing, and other measures for each service, along with an analysis of operational policies, functional requirements, patient care objectives, and growth assumptions. This picture will help in understanding overall trends, seasons of peak demand, and the link to operational goals. These must be tempered with an understanding of changing health care patterns.

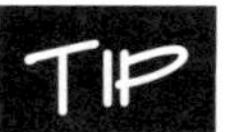

Computer simulations can provide a method for estimating the optimal space for operational performance. In areas where space and operating costs are high, where immediate access to services is critical, or where complex patient and material flows are involved, computer simulation models provide a mechanism for understanding interrelated spaces, staffing, and resource decisions. These models are generated based on census or workload data, staffing patterns, and physical layouts. Simulation can replicate variations in demand and space usage. They can also test potential design layouts for deficiencies and areas of congestion during peak census periods. Simulations can be modeled to project arrivals, treatment mix, and room use times. These models can then be used to estimate the need for patient care spaces. ■

Research the Guidelines and Requirements

As part of the data collection effort, organizations should research the state, local, and federal regulations that will impact the design, content, and layout of the facility. These regulations will vary depending on the state in which an organization is located and the type of facility being built. While the scope of this chapter does not allow for in-depth discussion on all the possible regulations and guidelines an organization must consider, following are several sources for information that organizations can and should consult:

State and local building codes. Many states and municipalities offer their building codes on their Web sites. Project teams should be familiar with these codes and have ready access to them.

American Institute of Architects (AIA). The AIA Guidelines for Design and Construction of Hospitals and Health Care Facilities are used as a reference code or standard by authorities in 42 states and several federal agencies when reviewing construction designs, plans, and completed health care facilities.[2] The 2001 edition is the most current; however, the guidelines are currently under review, and a new set should be available in early 2006.

Americans with Disabilities Act (ADA). The ADA prohibits discrimination and ensures equal opportunity for persons with disabilities in employment, state and local government services, public accommodations, commercial facilities, and transportation. It also mandates the establishment of TDD/telephone relay services. Some things that the ADA will specify regarding building design and content include the width of doorways, the presence of ramps in and out of a facility, the number of handicapped-accessible parking spaces, and so forth. A complete listing of the ADA requirements can be found at http://www.usdoj.gov/crt/ada/adahom1.htm.

Occupational Safety and Health Administration (OSHA). This government agency provides standards relating to the safety and health of workers. Requirements relate to several topics, including air quality, ergonomics, and safety. A comprehensive offering of OSHA's requirements can be found at www.osha.gov.

National Fire Protection Association (NFPA). This nonprofit organization provides scientifically based consensus codes and standards relating to fire safety. The NFPA's *Life Safety Code*®* (*LSC*) specifically addresses those construction features necessary to minimize danger to life from fire, including smoke, fumes, or panic.[3] More information on *LSC* compliance can be found in Chapters Three and Four.

American Society of Heating, Refrigerating, and Air-Conditioning Engineers. This organization offers standards and guidelines regarding heating, refrigerating, and air-conditioning systems.

Create a Facility Program

Depending on the size and scope of the project, a team may choose to create a preliminary facility program to determine a project's scope and anticipated facility needs. A preliminary facility program determines phasing and scheduling as well as estimated project budgets for early phases. Preliminary facility programs usually do not include a detailed space-by-space list of needs, but identify general departmental or functional area needs. A much more detailed development of a facility program occurs after a building project is initiated as a result of the master plan.

• *Life Safety Code*® is a registered trademark of the National Fire Protection Association, Quincy, MA.

SIDEBAR 2-6.
To Build New or Renovate

As planning progresses, organizations should evaluate whether to build new facilities or renovate existing ones. A wide variety of conditions will determine the viability of renovation, including the following:

- The amount and type of space available for renovation
- Mechanical and electrical system limitations
- Ability to work within the existing building's boundaries
- Location of columns and structural walls
- Location of vertical penetrations, such as mechanical shafts, elevators, and fire stairs

In some cases, organizations can renovate and convert existing space for less money than they can build new space. Often, however, renovation costs may exceed construction costs, due to unforeseen conditions, phasing, scheduling, or logistical complexities. Following are some issues to consider:

- Converting existing space to new functions frequently requires working with room dimensions, structural grids, and building configurations that force compromises to meet the needs and goals of the project
- Remodeling often triggers the need to upgrade existing structures to meet current building code requirements; this, in turn, increases construction costs
- Renovation can cause disruption of ongoing normal operations and require the relocation of services. Coordination of temporary relocation of services and the sequencing of events on the overall timeline may make remodeling more time consuming than new construction
- A renovation project may trigger correction of handicapped accessibility deficiencies in areas of the facility remote from the proposed renovation
- A partial renovation can result in the need for dual systems, which may increase operating costs and staff confusion. For example, although it is clear that digitized images are the wave of the future, when remodeling an imaging department, planning must accommodate both film and filmless systems

A preliminary facility plan generally includes the following elements:

- A tabulation of existing space
- A statement describing the general intent of the project
- The form of the project or what spatial/physical organization is required
- The long- and short-term cost/benefit implications of the project
- The time parameters for the project
- Future growth projections and space needs

A wide range of computer modeling tools and other guidelines are available to assist the project team with the creation of a preliminary facility program. Teams should be wary of using simple "rule of thumb" guidelines to estimate space needs. Estimating space based on inpatient beds or other simple statistics can easily overlook unique characteristics of an institution and the enormous changes occurring in health care.

Establish Functional and Physical Relationships

As facility programming progresses past the preliminary stage, different functional and physical relationships must be tested against the operational and physical constraints of the project. To visualize functional and physical relationships between project elements, project teams may want to develop diagrams. Generally, many diagrams will be produced that explore both inter- and intradepartmental relationships. Some may illustrate idealized conditions or optimum arrangements, while others may test desired relationships against physical constraints and design objectives.

The most elementary type of diagram is called a bubble diagram. Neither drawn to a particular scale nor proportionally accurate, bubble diagrams are used to illustrate process, organizational, operational, or functional relationships between defined elements. These functional diagrams are used to identify an optimum physical layout and organization of the spaces, people, and systems of the organization. This type of graphic is useful in understanding ideal relationships but is not useful in testing the layout and configuration of spaces or areas against actual building conditions.

Other Planning Considerations

Although examining different physical and functional relationships is important, other areas of the facility or campus should be considered during the programming process. These areas include the following:

Safety. As previously discussed, most errors in health care come from system issues, such as faulty procedures, inadequate processes, flawed equipment, or risks in the care environment. Organizations have an opportunity in the programming stage to focus on the safety of the building and how the building can promote safety throughout the organization. Conducting proactive risk assessments to identify safety issues and addressing identified risks is one way organizations can design with a safety focus. More information on designing for safety can be found in Chapter Three.

Equipment. Equipment planning is an essential and time-critical element of health facility planning and development. Selection of equipment, such as an x-ray or a PET scanner, will often affect the size and layout of a space. To determine the equipment space and design needs, an equipment list should be developed as part of the programming process. This will not only identify appropriate space considerations, but this list can be used as a preliminary pricing guide for the budget. More about equipment considerations can be found in Chapter Three.

Utilities. The project team should ensure that the project's utilities, including its mechanical, electrical, and air-handling systems, are determined early in the process and coordinated with existing systems. This is true regardless of whether the project is new, an addition, or a renovation. If the organization has not considered the cost, location, and functionality of utility systems early in the planning process, unpleasant surprises can emerge as cost estimates are developed. All too often organizations order equipment without considering the utilities required to run the equipment or keep it temperature controlled. This can result in utility costs that surpass the cost of the equipment. Consulting engineers can determine a project's utility requirements.

Create a Detailed Space Program

Organizations should outline the space needed to meet the project's goals and objectives. A detailed space program can be created by using likely scenarios and forecasted workloads to estimate key patient care spaces (patient beds, exam rooms, operating rooms) and develop estimates of the other space elements necessary to support these primary activity areas.

Detailed space listings are generated through working sessions with departmental representatives, tours of similar facilities, and examples from previous projects. A detailed space program usually involves a summary list that identifies department, building, and project area subtotals and totals. The list should also include a room-by-room space list organized by department, functional area, or physical component of the building or project. At minimum, this list should identify the name, number, and size of all rooms, spaces, areas, and departments to be included in the project.

Frequently, a narrative description is provided for all key spaces, which identifies what determines the size and character of each space. This detailed information may also be recorded on separate forms called room data sheets, which are developed for each room.

Finalize the Plan

The final step in the facility planning process requires the development of a definitive master plan. This involves the project team's review of the various options presented by the design team, with the most appropriate solutions being developed into a final conceptual plan that addresses all the planning goals and issues identified during preceding phases. Many organizations see the master plan as a living document that must be revisited, revised, and updated on a regular basis to respond to changing conditions. This plan, if developed properly, will be flexible enough to meet the evolving needs of the organization for several years. A well-crafted master plan is invaluable in preventing critical facility-related decisions, often with long-lasting consequences, from being made in an information vacuum.

Obtain a Certificate of Need

Certain states require organizations that are building or renovating a facility to obtain a certificate of need. This involves justifying to the state why the construction project is necessary—for example, why additional beds, services, or equipment is needed. This process allows states to provide a balance of services across health care organizations and ensures that each health care organization is adequately serving its community.

The federal government established Certificate of Need (CON) requirements in the mid-1970s, with states given the authority to administer this law. During the 1980s, the federal government dropped the requirement for CONs. Several states, however, held on to CON laws, although the trend is to discontinue them as the economics of health care become more controlling.

Although procedures vary from state to state, generally, projects exceeding a certain amount of total project cost must be reviewed through a CON hearing process. Often, specialized equipment or procedures, such as MRIs or an open heart surgery program, will require a CON as well.

Some states require that room-by-room (schematic) plans (*see* Chapter Three) and program justification be used for CON review. Most require only a room-by-room space program, block concept diagrams, and a cost estimate. Generally, these will be available at the end of the predesign phase. It is important to have a preliminary review with CON hearing staff early in the planning process and allow extra time in the schedule for the CON hearing process.

Phasing

As the planning phase draws to a close, organizations need to consider how the master plan or predesign will be implemented. Inevitably, implementation of most master plans must be accomplished in several phases, due to limits on available resources as well as operational and physical constraints. Phasing is a major planning factor and can have an immense impact on timing, schedule, and cost. It can also have a major impact on the care and comfort of patients and staff. Phasing must be a key consideration in the planning process. The first step in the phasing process should involve communication with staff and public that something major is about to happen. Subsequent steps will bring online new or revitalized services and spaces as recommended in the master plan or predesign phase.

Create a Schedule

As part of the planning process, the project team should estimate the length of time necessary to plan, design, obtain approvals, and complete construction. If everything goes well, the facility will take occupancy at the point forecasted by the timeline or Gantt chart.

To create a time line, the team must first identify and schedule the major milestones of a project. Typical milestones include points of organization input and key go/no-go decision points for the organization's board of directors.

Just as the entire project is broken into a sequenced series of milestones, each stage consists of a specific set of tasks or activities that should be defined and organized. It is necessary to identify each activity and to estimate task duration and interdependencies to establish an accurate overall timetable. It is wise to allow for some "float" time in the sched-

FIGURE 2-1. Bar Chart Project Schedule

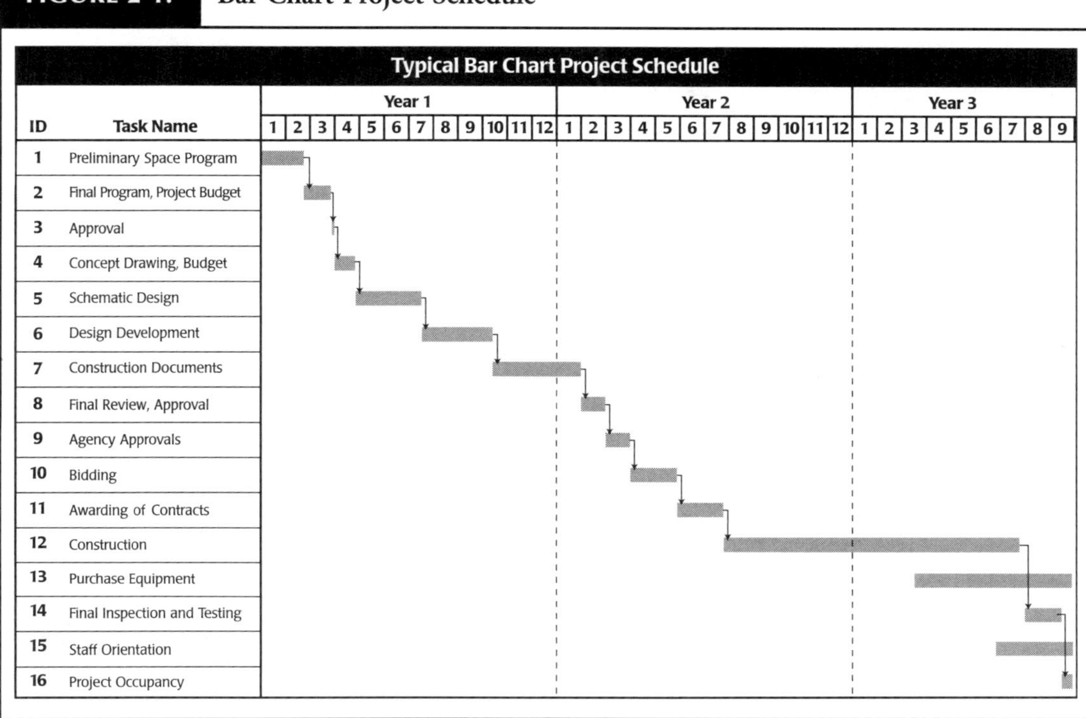

The bar chart compactly illustrates a total process. © 2006 Joint Commission Resources.

ule as a contingency for unforeseen events, such as delays in obtaining geological surveys, buying supplementary insurance, negotiating contracts, securing financing, and obtaining agency approvals.

After time estimates and relationships for each activity have been defined, several effective methods are available to determine the overall time line. The simplest employs a bar chart with a scale representing logical units of time, typically weeks for planning or months for large projects. The anticipated start date and duration of an activity are represented by the location and length of a bar extending across the graph. The bar chart has found wide acceptance, primarily due to its simplicity and its ability to illustrate a total process in compact form. Its major weakness is that it fails to identify those activities where completion or delay will have an immediate effect on the duration of the project. (*See* Figure 2-1 on this page.)

Another widely used technique for creating a time line is the critical path method. In the best-known version of this approach, each activity is represented by a line, while the completion of an activity or series of activities is represented by a circle or node. Activities are linked together in a sequence that shows the logical precedence and relationship of events. A given activity cannot start until all activities connected to the node preceding it are completed. The "critical path" is the set of activities that are linked such that a delay in any activity along the line will directly affect the project's completion date.

It is important for all team players to be familiar with the schedule and time line. Everyone should know specific deadlines for key events. As the plan is implemented, time estimates should be revised, as necessary, with an updated chart showing progress to date and remaining events.

Create a Budget

A project budget is more than just a construction budget. It includes all other costs associated with planning, design, and construction, such as equipment, furnishings, fees, interest, start-up costs, moving costs, land costs, contingencies, and so forth. Underestimating, or failing to identify and predict, total project-related costs is one of the biggest obstacles to successfully completing a project's design and construction.

Following are some critical costs that make up the project budget.

Construction cost. This is the most significant element of the estimated budget. Often, construction cost is 60% to 80% of total project implementation costs. Construction estimates are typically developed based on an approximated cost per square foot. Factors are applied to this estimate that reflect the geographic location, building occupancy classification, relative complexity of construction for each component of the project, and type of construction (for example, new or remodeled; wood, concrete, steel, or composite).

Anticipated equipment costs. These represent the second most significant element of the budget. Major medical equipment costs are among the most difficult to estimate in the early phases of a project. The specific services included in the project and the potential reuse of existing equipment can cause the total for equipment to range between 15% and 40% of the construction cost. Inventories of existing equipment, including an estimate of its remaining life expectancy, should be completed early in project development. Often, special equipment planning consultants are used for large projects, and several software programs are available to assist in developing equipment budget requirements.

Professional fees. This category covers professional services for all planning, predesign, design, and construction services, including consultants not traditionally covered by the basic architectural or engineering services. For example, the fees for construction management or a materials management consultant are not defined as basic architectural or engineering services.

Escalation fees. These fees come into play when there are unreasonable or unpredictable delays in the project or the general time frame is long. To account for escalation, construction projects are often estimated to the midpoint of construction, which means that the schedule must be known in detail prior to budgeting. A shared risk exists between the owner and construction team when setting an escalation factor. On a large project extending across a number of years, even a modest escalation factor of 3% per year can result in a significantly increased projection of construction cost.

Contingencies. The importance of budget contingencies cannot be overemphasized. Contingencies are a measure of uncertainty and will vary with each project. If an organization has an absolute limit on the dollars that can be spent on the project, the initial contingencies should be larger. If cost overruns are of little consequence, more dollars can be budgeted for the project itself and fewer for contingencies. Following are some contingencies for which organizations should plan:

Design contingency. Generally, a design contingency is established early in the predesign or design phase to cover unforeseen conditions. This contingency should be largest during the programming stage, but it can be reduced as design and documentation progress. Design contingencies for renovation projects vary considerably, depending on knowledge of hidden conditions such as asbestos, concealed mechanical and electrical systems, and building code changes.

Construction contingency. A construction contingency should be budgeted to cover field coordination and unanticipated conditions during construction. For new construction, a rule of thumb is to initially budget construction contingencies at 2% to 4% of construction cost; for remodeling 4% to 10% is usual.

Owner contingency. In addition to construction and design contingencies, the organization, or owner, should carry a contingency. Owner contingencies are often used for changes in project scope that occur after consultant bids are received. These can vary from 5% for new construction to 10% for smaller remodeling projects.

Contingencies reflect the imperfect and complex nature of the design and construction process and the lack of complete knowledge about conditions to be encountered when entering these phases. Denying the need for contingencies most often results in budget overruns, disappointment with the design and construction team, and possibly a reduction in project scope.

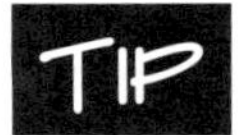

Architects, contractors, and construction managers who are familiar with health care construction should be the ones to estimate costs. Independent cost estimators may also be appropriate, particularly for large, complex projects. For final budgeting, the expertise of the estimator is particularly important. ■

Using a tool, such as a checklist, to generate an initial project budget can be helpful. Figure 2-2 on pages 43–44 is an example of such a tool.

Document the Plan

All project plans must be documented in a manner that is easily presented, understood, and used. For large, complex projects, organizations may wish to bind their master plan into a book that includes text narrative, tables, and drawings. This book should contain an executive summary that highlights key

FIGURE 2-2. Project Cost Checklist

Hospital Project Cost Checklist

Direct Owner Costs	
Administration, Financing, Accounting, Legal	$________
Insurance	$________
Development Studies and Reports	$________
Land Acquisition Costs	$________
Site Survey	$________
Geotechnical/Soils Report	$________
Field Trips	$________
A and E, Consultants' Reimbursable Expenses	$________
Fundraising Assistance	$________
Off-Site Traffic Mitigation Fees	$________
Off-Site Utility Projects and Mitigation Fees	$________
Construction Mock-up Allowance	$________
Permits and Plan Check Fees	$________
Testing and Certified Inspections	$________
Moving Expenses	$________
Financing Costs, Construction, and Long Term	$________
Subtotal Direct Owner Expenses	$________
Design and Construction Consultants	
Architectural/Engineering	$________
Specialty Consultants	$________
- Strategic Planning/Financial	$________
- Programming	$________
- Cost Estimating	$________
- Interior Design	$________
- Signage	$________
- Landscape	$________
- Transportation	$________
- Materials Management	$________
- Acoustical Engineering	$________
- Dietary	$________
- Telecommunications	$________
- Equipment	$________
- Vertical Transportation	$________
- Radiation Physics	$________
- Traffic/Parking	$________
- Environmental Impact	$________
- Americans with Disabilities Act	$________
Construction Management Services	$________
Subtotal Design and Construction Consultants	$________

Continued on page 44

FIGURE 2-2. Project Cost Checklist, continued

Furniture, Fixtures, and Equipment	
Medical Equipment	$________
Office Furniture and Furnishings	$________
Artwork	$________
Signage and Graphics	$________
Interior Landscape	$________
Telecommunications Equipment	$________
Computer and Data Systems Equipment	$________
Subtotal Furniture, Fixtures, and Equipment	$________
Construction Costs	
Demolition	$________
New Construction	$________
Renovation	$________
Site Work	$________
Off-Site Work	$________
Parking	$________
Landscape	$________
Subtotal Construction Cost	$________
Design Contingency	$________
Total Construction Costs	$________
Subtotal Project Cost	$________
Owner's Contingency	$________
Total Project Cost	$________

This useful tool can help generate an initial project budget.

goals, facts, issues, assumptions, facility needs, concepts, and master planning proposals. The executive summary should enable key decision makers to digest the most important information and make informed decisions without reading the entire document. The body of the document should be organized to reflect the key steps in the planning process and the findings that resulted from each step. These sections provide the substantiating evidence for the master plan proposals. Documentation of the master planning process may be located in an appendix and include such information as the work plan and schedule, meeting minutes, and background information.

Other ways to document the planning process include slides or other multimedia presentations, large presentation drawings of the plan proposals, and models that reflect the physical implications of the plan. These are useful for communicating the master plan to a broad range of constituencies in a wide variety of venues. Planning presentations often will be used to present to community groups, staff, board members, and the media. The ability to share the master plan with these groups is critical to its successful implementation.

SIDEBAR 2-7.
Tips for Success for Small Projects

The success of small projects hinges on the departmental representatives assigned to work with the project team. The ability to establish good communications between the representatives and the design team is critical. Both parties should learn each other's language and terms to ensure effective decision making. Special care should be taken to interpret and explain architectural terms and drawings.

For work on small projects, it is common for organizations to select architects and contractors who have worked with the organization before. An established record for communications, decision making, and execution can be critical when quick decisions are required with minimal owner input.

Some hospitals may also have the in-house capability to complete components of the planning and construction process. Careful coordination of tasks must be established to minimize potential conflicts between various in-house and contracted projects.

Small projects are subject to larger variations in cost than large projects. There are no small changes in scope and budget for these projects; any change is significant. A large project contingency (20% or more) should be maintained throughout the project.

SIDEBAR 2-8.
Tips for Success for Large Projects

For large projects to be successful, the organization must designate responsibility, authority, and time to an experienced administrator to manage the process. Meetings, newsletters, and other means of internal communication are keys to success in keeping communications flowing up and down the organization. Many organizations use an approach called "partnering" to coalesce complex teams of in-house staff and consultants.

Key Characteristics of Partnering

- Early identification of individual goals and resolution of conflicting goals
- Building lines of communication and mutual trust between project team members
- Setting common goals and project milestones relative to project scope, quality, and timing
- Establishing methods for later conflict resolution

Done well, partnering can offer considerable benefit by bringing teams together in a common focus. Partnering requires the use of outside consultants and a substantial investment of time by the organization and other team members, but the potential payoff includes improved communications, reduction of conflicts, and improved project coordination.

Keep a Balance

A well-built facility is determined by the interaction of three key factors: cost, quality, and quantity. In this triangle, when any part moves, the others are affected. Thus, all must be kept in balance. Keeping the balance of people, trust, dollars, and schedule in place is a juggling act. If any of these veers off course, the rest of the effort falls apart.

Planning can be an exciting adventure—fun and rewarding for all team members. A common, enthusiastic spirit and trust throughout will create a good result. A winning solution needs leadership that can provide a sense of passion and urgency throughout the process while nurturing and supporting the many participants and their constituents.

Trust and chemistry between client and design team are as important as the designer's skills. For a project to be successful, the team must have the ability to work closely together with mutual respect, to share the successes, and to work through the failures. Team leadership must recognize and rely upon the strengths of its participants, ensure open communication, and make timely decisions with respect to project scope and budget. This approach will best position the project for success.

REFERENCES

1. Siepel C., Hartwig P.: Collaborative design: Architects and contractors working together for client success in master planning. Paper presented at the ASHE International Conference and Exhibition on Health Facility Planning Design and Construction, Chicago, Mar. 7, 2005.

2. The American Institute of Architects: *Guidelines for Design and Construction of Hospital and Health Care Facilities.* http://www.aia.org/aah_gd_hospcons (accessed Jun. 6, 2005).

3. National Fire Protection Association: *NFPA 101: Life Safety Code®*. http://www.nfpa.org/aboutthecodes/AboutTheCodes.asp?DocNum=101 (accessed Jun. 6, 2005).

CHAPTER THREE:

Joint Commission Considerations for Planning and Design

PLANNING AND DESIGNING a health care facility is a multidimensional process. As discussed in Chapters One and Two, organizations must think about and plan for the type of building and building process they wish to have before breaking ground. In addition, organizations must also ensure that the facility design, structure, contents, and building process meet the requirements and standards of regulating and accrediting organizations, such as the Joint Commission.

An Overview of the Joint Commission Requirements

The Joint Commission has specific standards that address the planning, design, and construction phases. These standards address two major areas of design and construction:

Design and building layout. This includes designing for safety, security, emergency management, life safety, and infection control (IC). (Case Study 3-5 on pages 73–75 discusses how one organization incorporated all these considerations in its building process.)

The construction process. This process includes efforts to ensure that patient, staff, and visitor safety is preserved during construction. Requirements include a proactive risk assessment (including IC) and an assessment to determine required interim life safety measures (ILSM).

(*See* Sidebar 3-1 for a discussion of Joint Commission standards that address planning, design, and construction.)

Designing for Safety

The health care environment plays an important role in the safety of patients, staff, and visitors. For example, the layout of a patient room, the efficiency of a heating, ventilating, and air-conditioning (HVAC) system, and the design of a nurses' station can all affect the safety of care delivered by a health care organization.

Standard EC.1.10
(AHC, BHC, CAH, HAP, LAB, LTC, LT2, OBS, OME)
The organization manages safety risks.

Organizations have a valuable opportunity during construction and renovation projects to anticipate, address, and manage safety risks in a facility's design, programming, and layout. Some important actions

SIDEBAR 3-1. Standards That Address Planning, Design, and Construction

Safety Standard EC.1.10 requires organizations to manage safety risks. By incorporating a safety focus to the design and planning process, organizations can help manage safety risks through design.

Emergency Management Standard EC.4.10 requires organizations to address emergency management. Thinking about how a facility design can help address emergency issues, such as surge and emergency preparedness, can help an organization address emergency management.

Security Standard EC.2.20 requires organizations to address their security risks. Organizations can address this standard by thinking ahead of time about how building design can enhance security.

Life Safety Standard EC.5.20 requires all facilities, whether newly constructed, renovated, or existing, to comply with the *Life Safety Code*®* (*LSC*). Organizations must ensure that any new or renovated facilities meet the standards included in the *LSC*.

Infection Control National Patient Safety Goal 7 requires organizations to comply with all Centers for Disease Control and Prevention (CDC) hand hygiene guidelines, including providing conveniently placed alcohol-based hand rub dispensers and hand hygiene sinks. Organizations that consider how to best address IC during the design process can create a facility that helps prevent and control the spread of infection.

Proactive Risk Assessment Standard EC.8.30 requires organizations to conduct a proactive risk assessment to identify risks associated with air quality, IC, utilities, noise, vibration, and emergency procedures, and put controls in place to address those risks.

Interim Life Safety Measures Standard EC.5.50 requires organizations to protect building occupants, including staff, patients, and visitors, during the construction process by using ILSM to address lapses in *LSC* compliance.

* *Life Safety Code*® is a registered trademark of the National Fire Protection Association, Quincy, MA.

SIDEBAR 3-2.
Failure Mode and Effects Analysis

FMEA is a team-based, systematic, proactive technique used to identify issues and prevent problems before they occur. The FMEA technique is based on studied engineering principles and approaches to designing systems and processes. Following are the eight steps involved in the FMEA process:

1. Select a high-risk process and assemble a team.
2. Diagram the process.
3. Brainstorm potential failure modes and determine their effects.
4. Prioritize failure modes.
5. Identify root causes of failure modes.
6. Redesign the process.
7. Analyze and test the new process.
8. Implement and monitor the redesigned process.

SIDEBAR 3-3.
Human Factors

No matter how intelligent, skilled, or conscientious, individuals make mistakes, and certain factors enhance the likelihood of making mistakes in a complex environment such as health care. These factors are called human factors and can include the following:

- Limited short-term memory
- Being late or hurried
- Limited ability to multitask
- Interruptions
- Stress
- Fatigue
- Environmental factors, such as noise, light, and distractions[1]

that organizations can take to enhance safety include the following:

Consider potential safety risks and determine how design, layout, and construction can eliminate or reduce these risks. Such risks could include the following:

- Patient falls
- Medication errors
- Deaths of patients in restraints
- Inpatient suicides

Use a proactive risk assessment process, such as failure mode and effects analysis (FMEA), to identify places where safety could be compromised and design efforts to eliminate risk. FMEA is a proactive approach to systems improvement that involves anticipating areas where a system could fail and putting plans in place to prevent or mitigate the effects of those failures. The system in this case is the facility or building project. (*See* Sidebar 3-2, above.)

Address human factors, such as stress, fatigue, or interruptions, in design. (*See* Sidebar 3-3, above.) This could include standardizing room layouts so staff members do not need to acquaint themselves with the location of equipment, patients, and supplies every time they walk into a room. Standardizing reduces staff reliance on memory and can avert errors. Decentralizing nurses' stations can also address human factors issues. By putting nurses' stations closer to patients and including all necessary supplies in the work area, organizations can reduce staff fatigue and increase staff time with the patient.

Involve patients and staff. Organizations that partner with staff, patients, and families can gain a variety of perspectives on safety issues. Because staff members are on the "front lines" of care, they witness potential safety issues every day. Patients are on the receiving end of care and thus offer a different perspective of the safety and quality of care provided. Staff and patients can also give input to building design, layout, and construction issues.

Use the design and construction process to foster and enhance a culture of safety. By focusing on safety throughout the building process, organizations can further contribute to a safety culture. Open communication, proactive risk reduction, and patient and staff involvement will all help such a culture grow and flourish.

A focus on safety in the planning, design, and construction process involves a commitment from leadership, staff, and the project team. Without a group effort, safety issues can be overlooked or their importance minimized. Organizations should keep safety as a top consideration in all aspects of the building process. Case Study 3-1 beginning on page 50 illustrates how St. Joseph's Hospital incorporated safety into planning, design, and construction. For this organization, improving safety was more than just an important aspect of building design and construction; it was the main focus of the process.

Case Study 3-1. Focusing on Patient Safety During Design

St. Joseph's Hospital Takes a Proactive Approach to Addressing Safety Risks

St. Joseph's Community Hospital is an independent, nonprofit, 121-bed acute care facility located in West Bend, Wisconsin, near Milwaukee. Several years ago, St. Joseph's received the opportunity to build a new hospital. The organization recognized this as an opportunity to increase patient safety and promote a patient-safety culture by improving the traditional hospital facility design process.

Typically, hospitals are in a continuous cycle of remodeling and expanding their existing facilities to adapt to changing demands. St. Joseph's identified the need to develop a set of safety-driven design principles and design process recommendations that all health care organizations could use, whether they are building new facilities, remodeling, or expanding existing facilities.

A Learning Lab for Patient Safety

Inspired by the Institute of Medicine (IOM) report *To Err Is Human: Building a Safer Health System,* internal discussions at St. Joseph's in 2001 focused on how design of a new facility could affect patient safety. Initial discussions centered on whether to remodel the existing facility or build a new one. Hospital leaders determined that the costs to remodel and to build were comparable. In addition, building a new facility located near a major highway would provide convenient access to care for a growing population; allow the hospital to expand easily, if needed; and provide the opportunity to design around patient safety without the impediments of an infrastructure built in 1920.

It is widely acknowledged that the physical environment has a significant impact on health and safety; however, historically, hospitals have not been designed with the explicit goal of enhancing patient safety through facility design innovations.

Many considerations in facility design can influence the quality of care, such as light, noise, patient movement, patient visibility, and standardization. In researching how these considerations affected the quality and safety of patient care, St. Joseph's found a lack of available data. This led the organization to seek the advice of leaders in patient safety, quality improvement, and human factors. The belief was that an opportunity existed to collectively learn how a facility could be designed to improve patient safety.

In April 2002, leaders in systems engineering, health care administration, health services research, human behavior research, hospital quality improvement and accreditation, hospital architecture, medical education, pharmacy, nursing, and medicine participated in a conference, "Charting the Course for Patient Safety—A Learning Lab," sponsored in part by a grant from the University of Minnesota, Carlson School Program in Health Administration. The conference educated participants in facility design and safety, using lessons learned from the nuclear and transportation industries and spacecraft design.

The primary message of the learning lab was that safe hospitals could be designed by doing the following:

- Use a process that supports the anticipation, identification, and avoidance of failure
- Design against the latent conditions and active failures compromising physical and organizational defenses
- Create an organizational culture of safety[2]

Sessions directed participants to small work groups where they were led through a structured process established to develop recommendations that St. Joseph's could use to design a safe hospital. Participants were asked to consider designing around 10 specific precarious hospital events (*see* Figure 3-1 on page 51) identified earlier through a review of the Joint Commission's Sentinel Event Database and the safety topics of the Veterans Administration National Center for Patient Safety.

Each work group gave recommendations that led to the development of safety-driven design principles that guided the St. Joseph's design process (*see* Figure 3-2 on page 52). These principles focus on creating an environment that minimizes latent conditions and active failures in the health care facility.

Continued on page 51

Continued from page 50

Incorporating Safety into the Traditional Design Process

The traditional hospital design process requires that architects be given program objectives (role and program or master plan), which are then translated into room requirements (functional space program, from which department adjacencies (block diagrams) are created. After this preliminary information has been provided, room-by-room adjacencies are developed, and then a detailed design of each room is completed (schematic and design development). Architects then convert room-by-room design to construction blueprints that represent how individuals, equipment, and technology in hospitals will function together. Equipment and technology planning generally occur in the later stages of the design process. Typically, no discussions of patient safety or designing around precarious events are raised, creating an opportunity to repeat latent conditions in current hospital designs that contribute to adverse events or sentinel events. Human factors and the interface and impact of equipment, technology, and facilities are also not typically discussed or explored early in the process.

As a response to the learning lab, St. Joseph's made a decision to change the traditional hospital design process to incorporate the safety-driven design recommendations gleaned from the learning lab. Rather than just direct architects to design the new facility based on existing models, St. Joseph's focused the new development process on designing for the safety of patients.

In addition, the hospital approached the design process from a patient's perspective, from admission through discharge. This allowed St. Joseph's to identify areas of patient care that could be streamlined and develop initial adjacency recommendations. St. Joseph's conducted preliminary retreats and a technology fair to understand and prioritize facility features, technology, and equipment opportunities to meet safety-driven design principles, such as designing around precarious events. Participants included the design and construction team (architects, general contractors, and the owner's representative), hospital employees and physicians, and equipment and technology experts. The result was a matrix of prioritized opportunities of equipment, technology, and facility features that would maximize safety and quality within the proposed budget.

Additional changes to the traditional hospital design process included the following:

- Gaining input from a wide variety of persons, including learning lab participants, safety experts, patients and families, hospital employees and physicians, and community members

FIGURE 3-1. Precarious Events

St. Joseph's identified 10 specific precarious hospital events through a review of the Joint Commission's Sentinel Event Database and the safety topics of the Veterans Administration National Center for Patient Safety. Participants in the learning lab were asked to design around these events.

- Operative/post-op complications/infections
- Inpatient suicides
- Correct tube—correct connector—correct hole
- Wrong-site surgery
- Oxygen cylinder hazard
- Events relating to medication errors
- Deaths of patients in restraints
- Transfusion-related events
- Patient falls
- Magnetic resonance imaging (MRI) hazards

Source: St. Joseph's Community Hospital, West Bend, WI.

Continued on page 52

Continued from page 51

FIGURE 3-2. Facility Design Principles

These safety-driven design principles guided St. Joseph's design process.

Visibility of Patients to Staff
A window between the charting alcove and patient room will enhance visibility. Every patient care room should be wired for cameras and have proper lighting to allow staff to see patients consistently and accurately, day and night.

Standardization
Patient rooms should be truly standardized, including materials, gases, and head wall design.

Automate Where Possible
New technology has been shown to promote safety by adjusting for human limitations in memory and thought processes. Examples include bar-coding medications, electronic medical records, computerized provider order entry, centralized scheduling, and a tube system for delivery of materials.

Scalability and Adaptability
Forecasting the future is risky, and the facility must have the capability to easily accommodate, expand, and adjust to changes in technology and work processes. Facility design requires the flexibility to expand major services in the future and eliminate unsafe or outdated conditions with respect to ceiling height, wiring, tubing, lighting, door and hall width, building materials, and location.

Immediate Access to Information at the Point of Service
Critical information used for decision making should be close to the patient, with easy access at the point of service. Additionally, the design must accommodate an integrated information system to manage care processes from any point in the hospital. Lack of complete, accurate, and timely information creates errors in problem solving and can negatively impact the patient's condition and treatment plan.

Noise Reduction
Noise is correlated with fatigue and distractions that could lead to lapses and mistakes by staff. It is also correlated with poor sleeping patterns of patients, leading to slower immune system recovery. Examples to minimize noise include carpet, sound-absorbing ceiling tiles, and replacing the use of overhead paging systems with vibrating pagers.

Patients Involved with Care
Facility design should encourage patients and their family members to be involved with care. Empowering patients and families with the knowledge and encouragement to ask questions regarding treatment and medication will promote safety and teamwork. Spaces should be available for patients to be with their families.

Minimize Staff Fatigue
Fatigue is correlated with increased errors. Ways to minimize fatigue include reducing noise, allowing staff to sit as much as possible, having a "soft" floor, and minimizing distances staff must travel to provide patient care.

Use FMEA at Each Stage of the Design Process
Participants in the learning lab recognized FMEA as a basic design tool for patient safety. They recommended using FMEA at each stage of the design process to identify potential failures associated with proposed design solutions. The three key stages where FMEA should be used for design are adjacencies (block diagrams), schematics, and design development.

Design for Vulnerable Patients
Designing with patient interaction as the focal point provides opportunities to examine and change major organizational work processes, such as the movement of patients within the hospital and the admission and discharge of patients. When making design choices, the solution should work for the most vulnerable patient.

Human Factors Review
The impact of equipment/technology and facilities on human performance needs to be considered throughout the design process. Addressing human factors concepts, through such design principles as standardization and simplification, needs to be a priority throughout the design process.

Design Around Precarious Events
A review of the Sentinel Events Database of the Joint Commission and the Veterans Administration National Center for Patient Safety identified 10 specific precarious hospital events (see Figure 3-1 on page 51). Facility designs should anticipate and reduce the occurrence of these events as much as possible.

Source: St. Joseph's Community Hospital, West Bend, WI.

Continued on page 53

Continued from page 52

- Developing a checklist of the facility design principles to be used by the design teams (*see* Figure 3-3 on pge 54)
- Using FMEA at three design stages (adjacencies, schematic, and design development)
- Initializing mock-up and equipment planning at the onset of the design process
- Conducting focus group meetings and hospital staff and community surveys

A Team Approach to Design

Hospital leadership recognized that a cross-departmental team approach would be needed and formed the 11-member Facility Design Advisory Council (FDAC). Members of the council represented various departments within the hospital and included management, staff, and physicians. The council, led by the chief operating officer, was responsible for overseeing the design process and providing updated design information to hospital employees and administration.

St. Joseph's formed design teams for each department within the hospital. These department design teams, each ranging from 3 to 10 members, were put together by department managers. Each design team had multidisciplinary representation, including physicians from clinical areas. Each team, with the aid of the architects, was responsible for ensuring that the safety considerations of each facility design principle were met within its department. In addition, each team was required to complete a guiding principles checklist for its area and propose design recommendations to hospital leadership and the FDAC, which reviewed the design recommendations and worked closely with each department to finalize its plans. The FDAC's role was to ensure that the safety-driven design principles were met across and within departments in a standardized, uniform, and consistent manner.

St. Joseph's also periodically held retreats, including learning lab participants, content experts, the construction team, employees, managers, and the advisory council, to review progress in designing the new hospital to meet the safety-driven design principles.

Throughout the design process, the organization encouraged all hospital employees to share their opinions about existing safety concerns and give suggestions for improvements through e-mail, voice mail, a suggestion box, or by completing a staff survey. Either the department design teams or the FDAC reviewed these suggestions. The hospital frequently displayed updated information on the design process outside the hospital cafeteria and provided information in the weekly employee newsletter.

Community support was an important part of the design process. St. Joseph's formed focus groups to conduct community surveys to receive input into design from patients and families. Focus group suggestions on the patient room design, for example, led to an important relocation of the patient chair to allow an unrestricted path to the bathroom. St. Joseph's provided the community with regular updates on the facility design process and other efforts to improve patient safety through its community newsletters. In addition, the organization conducted several community town hall meetings on the building process.

Applying FMEA

To further ensure that safety was integral in the design and construction process, St. Joseph's brought in experts to educate representatives from the design and architect/construction teams on the use of FMEA. In hospital design, as in other industries, it is easier to fix potential failures during the planning stages than after construction has begun. Although using FMEA is very time consuming and often labor intensive, it can be very beneficial in identifying potential failures and developing innovative solutions associated with design considerations.

The design teams determined that the traditional FMEA approach was too complex for health care facility design and developed a modified approach[3]; a modified FMEA spreadsheet, in which failure occurrence and severity were scored as low, medium, or high, replaced traditional numeric scoring.

During the stage of the design process in which block diagrams of proposed adjacencies are determined, the hospital used FMEA to identify potential failures associated with proposed department adjacencies, by testing the adjacencies and other key processes when critically ill patients were moved to various departments (*see* Sidebar 3-4 on page 55).

Continued on page 54

Continued from page 53

FIGURE 3-3. An Excerpt from the Guiding Principles Checklist

The design teams use a checklist (excerpt shown here) to document use of the facility design principles shown in Figure 3-2.

Guiding Principles Checklist

☐ Visibility of Patients to Staff
Examples: Wiring for cameras, proper lighting, charting alcove with window
Comments: ____________________

Have you incorporated this principle into your department design?
☐ **Yes**
☐ No

☐ Standardization
Examples: Location of equipment, gases, and supplies, room design
Comments: ____________________

Have you incorporated this principle into your department design?
☐ **Yes**
☐ No

☐ Automate Where Possible
Examples: Bar coding medications, tube system/delivery of materials, nurse call system, dumb waiter/elevator adjacencies, centralized scheduling, bedside registration,
Comments: ____________________

Have you incorporated this principle into your department design?
☐ **Yes**
☐ No

Source: St. Joseph's Community Hospital, West Bend, WI.

According to the initial adjacency recommendations, the intensive care unit (ICU) was on a different floor than the emergency care center and radiology. As a result of applying FMEA to the proposed design, the design team relocated the ICU to be adjacent to emergency care, and designated the first floor a critical care level. Radiology, emergency care, surgery, the ICU, and the locked mental health unit were all located on the first floor to minimize the movement of vulnerable or critically ill patients. The behavioral health and ICU departments were adjacent to the emergency care center, with diagnostics and surgery immediately adjacent to the ICU and emergency care. In addition, St. Joseph's planned a rapid admissions area, with eight private rooms where patients could be observed and evaluated for up to 24 hours. Nonemergency patients begin in the rapid admissions area and have their lab work, x-rays, and other tests completed and recorded before being transported for treatment. For added safety, the design standardized all rooms in rapid admissions, ambulatory surgery, and emergency care in terms of layout and function to provide flexibility in use because patient levels vary in each department.

Planning for Equipment, Technology, and Mock-ups at the Onset of the Design Process

In keeping with the learning lab recommendations, planning for equipment, technology, and mock-ups started early. The equipment planner, architects, employees, physicians, contractors, and owner's representative all participated in this planning process.

The hospital held an on-site technology fair, where staff members had the opportunity to evaluate information systems and other technologies and generate ideas for application. St. Joseph's developed technology options to determine which systems could be implemented immediately or at the com-

Continued on page 55

Continued from page 54

pletion of the new facility and which could be acquired in the future. Priorities included using automated systems, when possible, to eliminate human error and having decision support and patient information available at the point of care. Initial technology plans included centralized scheduling, a nurse call system, pneumatic tube transport, and automated systems for the pharmacy, rapid admissions, and management of materials.

St. Joseph's then juxtaposed technology ideas with equipment needs and with potential facility design features that could maximize the safety-driven design principles, including precarious events. The design team created a matrix of specific ideas that would meet each design principle. The team then evaluated each idea to determine whether it could meet many or all of the remaining safety-driven design principles. After developing preliminary cost estimates, the hospital established priorities to implement these ideas, according to the extent to which the ideas would maximize safety by eliminating latent conditions and active failures. "We came up with $90 million in ideas for our $55 million dollar project, so prioritization was necessary but not impossible. There is a misperception that designing for safety costs more money. In fact, if organizations manage the money they have and prioritize how it is spent, they can still use safety design principles," says John Reiling, president and CEO of St. Joseph's Hospital.

Patient Rooms

Mock-up designs of patient rooms began immediately for the ICU, the medical/surgical floor, and the maternity ward. The designs used many different types of mock-ups, including two-dimensional and computer generated versions and actual physical construction. St. Joseph's constructed two mock-up rooms, one on the medical/surgical floor and the other in the maternity ward.

St. Joseph's then invited physicians, nurses, staff, patients, and family members to view and evaluate the rooms. The hospital placed suggestion forms in each room to encourage feedback. As a result of suggestions received from staff, the design team redesigned alcove storage, changed desk heights, and altered the configuration of the bathroom. The rooms went through multiple revisions of such important features as door sizes, locations of patient chairs, and lighting sources and locations.

SIDEBAR 3-4.
Failure Mode and Effects Analysis (FMEA): Analysis of the Movement of a Vulnerable (Critically Ill) Patient[3]

Using FMEA, St. Joseph's tested several scenarios in which a vulnerable patient was transported, including the following:

- A critically ill emergency department (ED) patient requiring radiology and direct admission to the intensive care unit
- A critically ill ICU patient in need of radiology and surgery
- An unstable medical/surgical patient being urgently transferred to the ICU
- A violent mental health patient brought to the ED and then admitted directly to the locked mental health unit

Through this analysis, the organization identified that the more frequently a patient must be moved, especially between floors, the greater the likelihood that errors could occur or equipment could fail, resulting in harm to a patient. In addition, ill patients need skilled staff to accompany them, therefore leaving key departments short staffed and creating the potential for errors and adverse events.

The patient rooms evolved from a "traditional" patient room to one based on the aforementioned safety-driven design principles. Each patient room in the new facility is a private room, allowing more space for staff to provide care and for family members who want to stay close to the patient. A small alcove adjacent to the room allows nurses to observe patients through a window without disturbing the patient's rest, creating greater visibility of the patient to staff and assisting the nurse in keeping patient information, supplies, and medication separate from those of other patients (*see* Figure 3-4 on page 56).

All rooms are standardized in layout, including location of supplies, equipment, and furniture. A cabinet or "nurse server" in each alcove holds the patient's

Continued on page 56

Continued from page 55

FIGURE 3-4. **Blueprint for a Patient Room**

This shows the blueprint for a patient room on the medical/surgical floor. ACC, (handicap) accessible; M/S, medical/surgical; PC, personal computer; TLT, toilet.

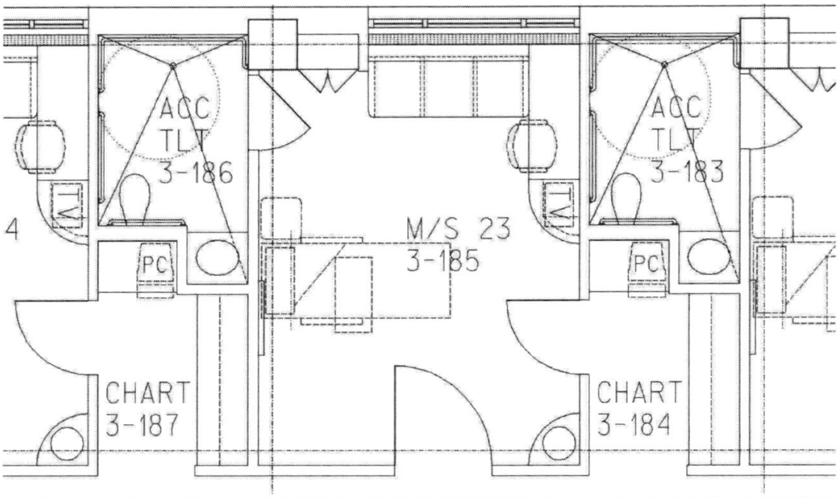

ACC
TLT
3-186
TV
4
PC
M/S 23
3-185
CHART
3-187
ACC
TLT
3-183
TV
PC
CHART
3-184

Source: St. Joseph's Community Hospital, West Bend, WI.

bar-coded medication (in a locked box) and all other supplies needed for patient care, allowing the nurse to remain in the room with the patient, reducing fatigue, and increasing time spent with the patient. The bathroom is located at the head of the bed, minimizing distance to the bathroom and ensuring that all patients have the opportunity to use handrail supports (*see* Sidebar 3-5 on page 57).

Evaluation

Ongoing evaluation of the existing facility and processes was critical to the design process. Identifying where errors occur and what latent conditions contribute to those errors assisted in identifying needed technology, improving processes, and creating safer, more efficient space in the new facility.

The organization conducted several Web-based conferences with learning lab participants to provide them with updates on the design process and gain feedback. The organization also periodically conducted retreats for members of the design teams and management. The retreats generated many ideas for discussion, including the following:

- Using infrared technology to reduce patient falls (the "electric eye" notifies the caregiver immediately when the patient sits up or moves toward the edge of the bed)
- Making sinks visible to patients and convenient to staff and providing pharmacy decision support software and electronic medical records
- Providing patient access to medication orders
- Wiring for future applications
- Monitoring a patient's cardiac rhythm across departments—that is, at any point in the hospital—without encountering any "dead spots," as some older facilities do

Challenges

St. Joseph's experienced three major challenges in designing for safety: gaining recognition of the need and opportunity to design a safer facility, maintaining focus on and commitment to the safety-driven design principles, and changing the traditional design process to incorporate the learning lab process recommendations.

Continued on page 57

Continued from page 56

Like many organizations, the leadership and staff at St. Joseph's did not initially understand the concepts of latent conditions and active failures and did not appreciate the prevalence of near misses and adverse events. "We initially believed that 'to err is human' happened in other states and facilities but not in Wisconsin or at St. Joseph's," Reiling said. "In addition, the external design team had to go through a culture change. The team members needed to recognize the opportunities for improved safety in designing a health care facility."

Change is difficult for many people; therefore, the need for consistency of purpose from management and the architects was essential. Requiring each design team to complete a detailed checklist forced each team to either incorporate a design principle into its proposed design or explain how it did not apply to its department.

Conclusion

By keeping safety at the forefront of design, St. Joseph's Hospital has created an environment where patient, staff, and visitor safety is preserved and maintained. But these efforts are not the end of St. Joseph's journey toward safety. Making St. Joseph's a safer place for patients and staff is an ongoing process that will continue well beyond the completion of the new facility. It will require hospital leadership, physicians, and staff to constantly focus on safety and will be accomplished only through a continuous cycle of evaluation and improvement of the facility, equipment, technology, and processes. The organization designed the new hospital with maximum adaptability and flexibility in mind, to accommodate changes and provide for future growth. The entire facility can be expanded with minimal disruption by expanding the wings and adding a fourth patient care floor.

SIDEBAR 3-5. Safety Features of a Patient Room

- Standardization in room size/layout
- In-room sink to allow physician/staff hand washing in patient view
- Charting alcove with window to increase patient visibility for nurses, physicians, and staff
- Private room to provide privacy
- Close proximity between bed and bathroom to reduce the potential for patient falls
- Bedside computers to allow patient access to records (for example, scheduled medication or other treatments prescribed) and thereby increase involvement with care. They also allow nurses or other staff to double-check medication or other scheduled treatment before administration.
- Oversized windows to increase natural light and provide a "healing" view
- Ceiling heights and room size to allow adaptability/suitability
- Sitting area and guest foldout bed to encourage family support
- Noise reduction, through use of low-vibration steel and special noise-absorbing ceiling tiles and elimination of overhead paging
- Improved technology, including electronic medical records, computerized physician order entry, and advanced nurse call system (including wireless phones)
- Use of infrared technology to reduce the potential for patient falls

Worker Safety

Although most of the Joint Commission's focus on safety is related to the safety of patients, EC.1.10 does require organizations to preserve the safety of staff as well. Many of the previously mentioned safety-improvement strategies will enhance the safety of staff while enhancing patient safety. In addition, as discussed in Chapter One, organizations can specifically address worker safety issues by considering ergonomic issues. Designing facilities to limit staff injury, such as back injuries resulting from improper patient lifting, can enhance the safety of staff and improve their morale, satisfaction, and ability to provide comprehensive care. Case Study 3-2 beginning on page 58 describes how one organization improved the safety of staff by engineering out areas of risk.

Case Study 3-2. Developing Systems to Prevent Worker Injury

Seattle Children's Hospital Addresses Ergonomic Design

Back injuries can be the most severe and costly musculoskeletal injuries that health care organization staff can experience. Seattle Children's Hospital and Regional Medical Center, a pediatric referral center for the states of Washington, Alaska, Montana, and Idaho, was concerned about the number of back injuries that were occurring in its facility. "These types of injuries often are the most costly in terms of money and resources. In addition, they have the potential to end a health care worker's career, although most will fully recover. As an organization, we wanted to minimize the likelihood of these injuries, so as to preserve the health and safety of our staff," says Therese Bovee-McKelvey, R.N., M.N., C.O.H.N.-S., manager for Occupational Health Services at Seattle Children's Hospital.

Immediate Actions to Address Ergonomic Issues

Seattle Children's began its efforts to reduce worker injury by tracking all worker injuries and looking at the data. As with other organizations, back injuries had the largest impact on the organization's resources. Many of these back injuries occurred as a result of lifting or transporting patients. To address this issue, the organization developed a policy, with input from nursing directors and nurses, that specifically relates to "patient handling," which includes transfers, lifting, repositioning, and assisting.

This policy requires staff to take the following actions:

1. Evaluate the risk/hazard of the transport or lift situation
2. Get assistance before attempting to transfer, lift, or reposition a patient
3. Don't assume that assistance is not needed. Even if a patient is small, staff is instructed to get assistance for transporting or lifting. Many times patients can move during the transferring process, causing the staff member to twist, stretch, or reach in an unnatural way; this can result in injury. In addition, a pediatric patient may be small but equipment can be the problem, such as a bed or stretcher and one or two IV poles.

Seattle Children's educated staff on the policy and also provided training for staff on the proper way to lift, transport, and reposition patients.

In addition to addressing the risks associated with patient transfer, Seattle Children's implemented strategies to reduce safety risks in other day-to-day staff activities. For example, the organization replaced carpets with vinyl flooring, where possible. Vinyl offers less resistance than carpet and thus equipment, such as IV poles, are easier to move and control, reducing the hazard for injury.

Seattle Children's also examined the wheels on its portable equipment. Where possible, the organization put larger, fatter wheels, which were less likely to get stuck, on equipment. One important area the organization looked at was equipment maintenance. Proper maintenance can prevent equipment from breaking, malfunctioning, or seizing up—issues that can sometimes cause injury.

Addressing Other Types of Lifting. Staff members can injure themselves lifting other things besides patients. For example, much of the stock in the pharmacy arrives in heavy, awkward boxes on pallets. Seattle Children's, through the help of an ergonomics consultant, designed a conveyer system/palette lift that allowed staff to interact with stock at an appropriate height. A similar system was also used in the mail room.

Addressing Ergonomic Issues in Design and Construction

In 2003, Seattle Children's had the opportunity to consider ergonomic issues in the design of its new inpatient nursing unit. To ensure that worker safety was addressed in the building, the organization gathered data and involved staff early in the process. The organization looked at a variety of areas in design to ensure worker safety, including equipment, room layout, and staff workstations. "We requested that the design team work with an ergonomics consultant to help ensure the ergonomically appropriate design of the facility. A consultant can offer a different perspective. He or she can consider the needs of all types of people and the organization's history with ergonomic issues," Bovee-McKelvey says.

Some of the actions taken by the organization to address worker safety in design include the following:

Continued on page 59

Continued from page 58

- *Installed ceiling lifts in patient rooms.* These types of lifts include a patient sling and a motorized pulley system or motorized unit that helps with lifting. They can be ceiling mounted or freestanding, depending on the needs of the organization. In addition to minimizing worker injury, ceiling lifts optimize space use because they take up no floor space. The decision to install ceiling lifts in the new facility was made by a multidisciplinary group, consisting of facilities, nursing, and design team personnel. The organization wanted lifts that were easy to use, discouraged patient play, were safe, and had washable patient slings, to meet the organization's infection control requirements. Vendors demonstrated the equipment to the organization, and the organization chose a type of lift based on the aforementioned needs and budget. The hospital installed the ceiling lifts in a selected number of rooms designated by the inpatient nursing units and rehab. In designing these areas, the organization made sure that a bathroom was placed in every patient room. Later in the mock-up phase, the group determined that for rooms with ceiling lifts the tracking area needed to be extended into the bathroom to allow transfer of patients from room to bathroom and back.

- *Designed patient rooms to be ergonomically correct.* Seattle Children's was careful to design the room so that staff would not need to bend or stretch to reach items. The hospital solicited the input of nursing and respiratory therapists to address ergonomic issues, such as where to put outlets and supplies.

- *Designed workstations to be ergonomically correct.* The organization included sit and stand workstations in its new facility. These workstations offer staff members the opportunity to sit or stand during their work. "Mock-ups were done for sit/stand models and for unit coordinator stations. Mock-up evaluations allowed us to make changes where needed and at a time when least expensive. These mock-ups resulted in redesigning workstations to give nurses more room and work surface space," says Bovee-McKelvey. The organization also lowered the transaction counters at unit coordinator stations so that unit coordinators did not need to crane their necks to see people approaching the counter.

- *Trained staff members on how to adjust their work space to address their ergonomic needs.* "We worked with the vendor to provide equipment-specific training for ceiling lifts prior to moving patients into the area. Before this, a new administrative building was completed, which introduced new workstation designs and layout, so ergonomic classes were given to prepare staff to make the most of the new designs and equipment. We also offered annual training on ergonomic issues to reinforce their importance," Bovee-McKelvey says.

By using these design strategies in the new building, along with the policies and procedures mentioned earlier, Seattle Children's has seen a decrease in the number of staff injuries. "The best way to save money on ergonomics is to build it into the design. It costs a lot more money to remake or remodel a bad ergonomic design than to get it right the first time. The money you save will be from not having to remodel and avoiding ergonomic injuries and claims," says Bovee-McKelvey. Partnering with staff early in the process can not only identify issues that need to be addressed but can develop organizational awareness of ergonomic issues.

CASE AT A GLANCE

■ Main challenge
To reduce back and other worker injuries throughout the organization.

■ Issues
Improper lifting and transferring of patients can lead to worker injury. Other activities, such as stretching, bending, and reaching, can also lead to injuries.

■ Solutions
The organization implemented a new patient transferring and lifting policy, educated staff on the policy and appropriate ways to lift and transfer patients, and considered ergonomic issues in the design of its new facility. One specific design element it implemented was ceiling-mounted patient lifts.

■ Outcomes
Through its new policy and the design strategies used in the new building, Seattle Children's decreased the number of worker injuries.

Designing for Emergency Management

On December 26, 2004, health care organizations across the world received a vivid reminder of how an ordinary day can quickly become extraordinary. In the hours and days after powerful tsunamis, caused by an earthquake under the Indian Ocean, hit the shores of India, Indonesia, Sri Lanka, Thailand, and the Maldives, thousands of survivors rushed to receive medical treatment. This disaster graphically illustrates that no country is immune to emergencies and that front-line providers, including hospitals and other health care organizations, must be prepared to respond.

Standard EC.4.10
(AHC, BHC, CAH, HAP, LAB, LTC, LT2, OBS, OME, HDS)
The organization addresses emergency management. (CAH: Corresponds to COP 485.623 (c)(3) and (c)(4))

Standard EC.4.10 requires organizations to address emergency management. One of the ways organizations are required to do this is by creating an emergency management plan. This plan must identify mitigation, preparedness, response, and recovery strategies. Mitigation activities are those that lessen the severity and impact of an emergency. This is the aspect of emergency management planning that can be addressed through proper facility design. For example, by designing a building to handle patient surge situations, organizations can lessen the severity and impact of the emergency. Some issues to consider when designing for emergency management include the following:

Patient flow. This involves how patients will arrive at, enter, move through, and exit the facility in a safe orderly manner. During an emergency the volume of patients will increase and so will the level of tension. Individuals may be rushed or panicked. Design should streamline patient flow to ensure the consistent movement of patients through the facility. In addition, the building should be designed so emergency medical professionals, such as paramedics, enter the building through a different entrance than ambulatory patients. This prevents ambulatory patients from getting in the way and also from seeing victims with more serious health issues.

Security. During an emergency, organizations will need to effectively control the entrance and egress activities. Most likely, organizations will need to lock down a site to maintain order and security.

Wayfinding. Many people will enter a health care facility during an emergency, and most of them may never have been in the facility before. Organizations should have effective wayfinding systems to guide patients where they need to go. If patients are being asked to go different places than they normally would when visiting the hospital, temporary wayfinding systems should be established to guide patients safely to the appropriate location.

Decontamination. Depending on the type of emergency, an organization may need to decontaminate patients. This could involve showers and negative pressure rooms. Organizations should consider how to keep "dirty" patients away from "clean" ones and how to prevent the spread of infection. An organization may need to shut off the emergency department (ED) from the rest of the facility in certain situations. Organizations should ensure that this capability is built in during design.

Parking. An emergency typically creates an influx of vehicles, including emergency vehicles, personal vehicles, supply delivery vehicles, and so forth. Organizations should consider parking logistics and design parking structures to accommodate a surge in vehicles.

Convertability. The design team should consider developing spaces that can be converted, during an emergency, into patient care, triage, or holding areas. Such spaces could include ambulatory surgery suites, office space, or meeting rooms. Organizations may want to design some of these rooms to be close to the ED so staff does not need to travel far. On the other hand, if they are preparing for a biological emergency where cross-contamination could occur, organizations may want to design convertible areas far away from the main hospital building.

By considering these issues before an emergency, organizations can ensure safety and appropriate, high-quality care during an emergency. If the building project includes an ED, organizations should consider hiring an architect who specializes in emergency room design.

In addition to designing existing facilities to handle surge situations, organizations may want to consider designing a surge facility that operates only during emergencies. Case Study 3-3 on pages 61–62 describes some creative ways to design such facilities.

Case Study 3-3. Designing for Surge

Texas A&M University Students Create Solutions

In response to the events of September 11, 2001, the Texas A&M University System Health Science Center, Office of Homeland Security, charged the students of the Texas A&M University College of Architecture with researching ideas and architectural concepts for self-sustaining surge hospitals. A surge hospital is designed to respond to surges of large numbers of patients due to an emergency. Such a hospital would take over in the event an existing hospital was unable to treat patients, due to such conditions as inaccessibility, destruction, or being at or over capacity.

A surge hospital is a self-sufficient facility that must function as its own city during a surge situation. Some issues the students considered when designing their surge hospital included the following:

How is the surge facility used during nonsurge situations? It would be a waste of resources to have a facility sit empty until an emergency occurs. Surge hospitals should have a dual use or multiple uses.

Power sources. Surge facilities must have multiple backup power sources, in case of a power failure.

Storage. Facilities must be able to store medical supplies, food, water, and extra beds. The students needed to consider the quantity of supplies, food, and water that would be kept on hand at all times, and what quantity would need to be brought in during the emergency. For those supplies kept on hand, the students had to consider how often supplies, food, and water needed to be cycled to stay fresh.

Location. The location of a surge hospital must be convenient, easily accessible, and able to handle an influx of patients. Students had to consider the flow of traffic coming and going from the facility, as well as address how emergency rescue vehicles, such as helicopters, ambulances, and fire trucks, would arrive at the scene. Students also had to consider parking issues.

Security. The students had to consider how patients and staff would be protected within the facility. This included determining the need for a fence or some sort of barrier system, the appropriate number of entrances and exits, and the ability to lock down the facility, if necessary. Many students incorporated a secured narcotic storage area to their designs. This could prevent dangerous drugs from getting into the wrong hands.

Information/communication centers. The surge facility needs to have space for an emergency command center that would coordinate communication with community leaders, the fire department, the police department, other hospitals, patients, families, and staff.

Family and friend accommodations. These are accommodations for patient's friends and families who do not require medical attention, but who want to stay near the patient. The students designed facilities so that staff could quickly separate people who needed treatment from people who did not. Color-coded wayfinding systems were used to help people move through the facility in an orderly fashion. Depending on the situation, surge hospitals can also provide shelter, food, and water for people displaced from their homes by disasters.

Waste and laundry. An emergency is going to generate a lot of these two things. The students needed to consider how to effectively handle hazardous materials and waste, as well as nonhazardous waste, and how to foster the quick and efficient turnaround of laundry. Some students addressed the laundry issue by suggesting the surge facility pair up with a Laundromat.

Staff. Because the surge hospital is taking over from the existing facility, one has to assume that all or some of the staff will not be able to staff the surge facility. For example, if the existing hospital is operating at maximum capacity, it will not be able to share any staff with the surge facility. Students had to consider where new staff would come from. Some suggested using retired medical personnel from the community, alternate shift personnel, and personnel from nearby behavioral, long term care, or ambulatory care facilities.

Decontamination. Students had to allow space in their design for a decontamination area. They needed to control entrance and egress to the build-

Continued on page 62

Continued from page 61

ing to prevent cross-contamination. Some students used outdoor spaces that could quickly be covered and converted into decontamination spaces.

Although the ideas that came from the project are just ideas, some of them offer tremendous possibilities for improving an organization's emergency response. Following are some of the ideas:

Dual-use facilities. As mentioned previously, surge facilities must have other uses besides just responding to a surge situation. A dual-use facility serves another purpose for most of its existence but can be converted quickly into a surge facility. Some ideas for dual-use facilities included a wellness center, a hotel, a clinic, a gym, and a retirement center. All these facilities could have a nearby park with baseball fields that could serve as a helicopter landing area. For facilities such as hotels and retirement centers, the students considered what would happen to the individuals displaced by the emergency (for example, hotel guests or long term care residents).

Medical mobile units. These are large trucks that tour rural areas and provide health care services, such as imaging, outpatient surgery, women's health, or wellness care. Depending on the day, a particular unit could be in any one of the rural areas. During a surge situation, the multiple trucks from surrounding areas could be called to a main site to serve as the surge facility. For example, the trucks may park in the parking lot of a high school or community center. Mobile medical units not only address emergency management, but they also address rural health issues by bringing high-quality health care to rural areas.

Thursday hospital. This type of facility combines the concepts of a dual-use facility with a mobile medical unit. Like a dual-use facility, the Thursday hospital is not a surge facility all the time. It has multiple uses, depending on the day. For example, on Monday it could be a courtroom, on Tuesday a gym, on Wednesday a boys and girls center, and on Thursday a hospital. The mobile medical units arrive on Thursday to provide health care services. Because the site is multifunctional, it would house only the bare minimum of health care supplies and accommodations. The vans would supplement materials provided by the facility to make a complete medical unit. As in the previous example, multiple medical units would arrive during a surge and partner with the "Thursday" hospital to make a complete surge facility.

While the creativity of these ideas can really cause an organization to think, the most important aspect of emergency planning is the planning. "We learned that organizations should plan now for emergencies and have multiple backup plans. All the structures in the world won't help if emergency response has not been planned," says Allison Prehn, an architecture student at Texas A&M.

Not every organization will need a surge facility. A good hazard vulnerability analysis should help an organization determine if such a facility is warranted and what kind would be appropriate.

CASE AT A GLANCE

■ **Main challenge**
To create design options for a surge facility.

■ **Issues**
In preparing for emergency management, organizations may want to consider designing a facility that could take over during an emergency, when the existing facility is unable to treat more patients. Organizations should consider location, size, staffing, and patient flow issues in design.

■ **Solutions**
Architecture students created many design options, including the dual-use facility, mobile medical units, and the Thursday Hospital.

In 2003, Toronto hospitals experienced a surge of infectious patients as a result of the SARS epidemic. Case Study 3-4 on pages 63–66 describes how the organizations had to improvise to avoid having the entire facility contaminated. Organizations can learn from these strategies and incorporate proactive ideas to address surge situations.

Case Study 3-4. What Toronto Hospitals Learned from SARS

Facing Down a Serial Killer

What became a rampage started off innocently enough in November 2002. Striking first in China's Guangdong Province, the killer masqueraded as just another case of atypical pneumonia. But the outbreak spread with terrifying rapidity, and by the time it had run its course eight months later, what would become known as Severe Acute Respiratory Syndrome (SARS) would afflict approximately 8,500 people around the world and kill more than 900.

Outside Asia, Canada was the country hardest hit by SARS. From March 2003 to July 2003, Canadians counted 438 probable and suspected cases of SARS, with 44 deaths from the disease. Most of the SARS cases and all the deaths occurred in and around the Toronto area, where more than 100 health care workers contracted SARS and 3 died.

Canada's National Advisory Committee (the Canadian counterpart of the U.S. Centers for Disease Control and Prevention charged with investigating the SARS outbreak) cited several deficiencies in the response to the disease by the clinical and public health systems. Among these was the lack of surge capacity, meaning the ability to handle an influx of patients. The experiences of two Toronto hospitals highlight the importance of facilities management in establishing and maintaining surge capacity—an increasingly critical component of an emergency management plan and one that is required for Joint Commission–accredited hospitals in the United States by standard EC.4.10.

North York Hospital—Ground Zero in the SARS Wars

Toronto's North York General Hospital is a 434-bed facility positioned at the epicenter of the second phase of the SARS outbreak. What came to be known as SARS I lasted from March 27 to April 15, 2003. At the end of five weeks, health officials were catching their breath on the assumption that the disease had run its course, and the hospital had begun resuming its services at near-normal levels. That's when the disease struck again in the form of SARS II, which for this hospital lasted from May 23 to August 19, 2003.

"We went from 30 SARS patients in the first wave to more than 90 during the second wave," says Bonnie Adamson, president and CEO of North York General Hospital. Even though staff did not contract the disease during SARS I, 44 staff became ill during SARS II. Among the Canadians who died was a North York General Hospital nurse who had been caring for patients later found to have had SARS.

As the scope of the outbreak broadened, North York General Hospital had to expand its SARS capacity—and do it fast. Hospital management reacted almost overnight. Fortunately, North York was nearing completion of a new hospital facility, which included a 24-bed ICU and new inpatient units. So hospital management fast-tracked completion of the ICU in that new building and thus was able to open more than 70 beds in the ICU and in two units dedicated to SARS patients. Most important, all 70 beds had the all-important negative air pressure (*see* Sidebar 3-6 on page 64). To redeploy its resources to fight SARS, North York General Hospital closed the emergency department (ED) and the obstetrics unit, restricted elective surgeries, and shut down many of its clinics.

Because code orange was declared for the province, North York stopped all ambulatory activity. Patients were then redirected based on the necessity of their situation. According to Susan Kwolek, vice president of quality and corporate performance at North York, "Any [ambulatory] activities that were elective, such as visits to clinics, were considered discretionary and therefore canceled." However, any nonelective ambulatory activities, such as prenatal care and oncology visits, were assessed on a case-by-case basis. North York notified patients with appointments of any cancellations or new arrangements with clinics in offices outside the organization. "Other hospitals were in the same situation, so we could not use partnerships or alliances," Kwolek says.

By the time SARS II struck, North York's focus was on preventing health care workers and other patients from contracting the disease. That meant

Continued on page 64

Continued from page 63

isolating SARS units from the rest of the facilities while still providing needed hospital services, such as housekeeping, dietary services, maintenance, and more. Management and clinical staff worked closely with the building services and facilities management staff. One example was a policy inaugurated by the hospital of checking for negative air pressure three times a day and reporting results to reassure staff. Finally, in early August 2003, North York was able to declare itself free of SARS patients.

Sunnybrook & Women's—Leaders in the SARS Battle

One of Canada's largest health care facilities, Sunnybrook & Women's (S&W) is a 1,400-bed tertiary/quaternary center that is an amalgam of three separate hospitals located around Toronto. During SARS I, S&W screened thousands of staff and visitors daily for SARS and managed more than 70 inpatients, the largest volume of in-hospital SARS patients outside mainland China. Additional pressures were placed on S&W as other facilities closed due to SARS outbreaks.

As the largest trauma center in the country, S&W treated almost all the trauma patients in the greater Toronto area and saw a significant increase in the number of ED visits. The hospital's director of facilities services, Harry Taylor, recalls, "When SARS first hit, we knew very little about the disease. But it quickly became evident that our number one priority had to be creating negative pressure rooms." The hospital chose to dedicate a general medicine floor as a SARS unit and almost overnight turned the 22 rooms in that unit into negative pressure rooms. In newer isolation rooms, an automatic alarm indicates when the room loses negative pressure. But S&W couldn't afford the time to buy and install those monitoring units. So facilities engineers set up a testing program to make sure the rooms were in fact staying negative. "Each day our technicians performed smoke testing to show which way the air was flowing," says Taylor. "And each day they would see smoke disappear underneath the door of the patient rooms, indicating that all was well with the negative pressure."

In their concern about ensuring negative air pressure, S&W filtered the exhaust through high-efficiency particulate air (HEPA) filters that would screen out any harmful elements. The hospital purchased 22 portable units from a supplier in Quebec. "When we told them how critical the situation was," Taylor says, "they shipped the filters overnight, and we had them installed in less than 24 hours."

SIDEBAR 3-6. Saving Lives Through Negative Pressure

In normal rooms, the pressure of air in the patient's room is greater than the pressure of the air circulating in the hallway. So opening the door to a patient room allows air from that room to enter the hallway. But with negative pressure rooms, air pressure in the corridor is stronger than in the patient room. So when the door opens between the two areas, air from the corridor enters the patient room. Negative pressure does the following:

- Prevents infected air from a patient room from entering the hallway
- Exhausts air from a patient room to the outside, rather than to the corridor

The hospital was also the first health care facility in Toronto to create a SARS assessment unit where symptomatic community residents could come to the ED to be evaluated for possible SARS. To accomplish this, S&W set up nearly 5,000 square feet of space at its Women's College Ambulatory Care Centre about five miles from the main campus and staffed it with doctors, nurses, and security officers. This was an important strategy to keep potential SARS patients away from the main facility.

The Role of the Facility Manager

Taylor points out that, in coping with an emergency such as SARS, facilities managers play a vital role and can draw on a wealth of resources. In addition to their own staff, they have access to engineering groups, suppliers, and peer groups at other hospitals.

Taylor's advice to other facilities management people who might someday face a similar challenge: "Be a strategic resource for your organization and work

Continued on page 65

Continued from page 64

closely with your senior leadership team. Educate people on the technical aspects of the building environment. Help in the development of tactical strategies, and then execute your plans quickly."

U.S. hospitals following Joint Commission emergency management standards (EC.4.10) will be completing a hazard vulnerability analysis to identify in advance potential emergencies that could affect the need for their services or their ability to provide those services. This would be an opportunity to set up preestablished supplier relationships for the identified vulnerabilities.

SARS also allowed S&W to test its ability to respond to a large-scale emergency. "S&W did an amazing job in pulling together," says Taylor. "It was stressful for everyone in the hospital, but the 400 people on our facilities management team—plant operations, environmental services, security, and our parking and transportation group—never hesitated for an instant to do what was needed. In fact, some of our people volunteered to take on tasks that would require them to be quarantined at work and at home."

Recommendations

Following is a list of recommendations for hospital facilities managers culled from suggestions by Kwolek and by Lucy Brun, a Toronto area health care and infectious disease expert:

- Provide sufficient surge capacity to address emergencies
- Reduce the number of entry/exit points to the facility; control access via cameras and swipe cards
- Separate the hospital's "mission critical" departments and access to these areas
- Increase the number of isolation rooms that include technique anterooms and three-piece washrooms
- Implement mechanical and ventilation systems to support isolation and separation of air intakes and exhaust
- Provide adequate individual space per patient; for example, more than four feet from one patient/visitor face to the next patient/visitor face
- Keep an adequate supply of personal protective equipment (face masks, gloves, gowns, and so on) on hand at all times and make sure that those supplies are readily available
- Clean patient units on every shift
- Clean all facilities and equipment that are in common use; for example, nursing stations, computer keyboards, telephones, and so on
- Use basic infection control methods as outlined in Joint Commission standards for the Surveillance, Prevention, and Control of Infection, in the applicable accreditation manual
- Consult the Web site of the Centers for Disease Control and Prevention at http://www.cdc.gov/page.do, which has a section devoted to SARS at http://www.cdc.gov/ncidod/sars/ and at http://www.cdc.gov/ncidod/sars/guidance/I/index.htm

SIDEBAR 3-7. The Other Diseases

Public health officials consider SARS to be the first severe and readily transmittable disease of this century. But many other diseases have been identified in recent decades. Organizations will want to consider these in their emergency management plans. Among them are the following:

- Bioterrorism (for example, chemical warfare, smallpox)
- Dengue fever
- Avian flu
- Malaria
- Methacillin-resistant staphylococcus aureus
- Norwalk
- Vancomycin-resistant enterococcus
- Chicken pox
- Ebola
- Influenza
- Meningitis
- Multiresistant tuberculosis
- Other respiratory viruses (for example, RSV, para-influenza)
- West Nile virus

U.S. Hospitals Prepare for the Future

Health care organizations in the United States are benefiting from Canada's experience. Skip Gregory, bureau chief of the Office of Plans and Construction at Florida's Agency for Health Care Administration,

Continued on page 66

Continued from page 65

reports that the agency is currently investigating how to expand the surge capacity of Florida hospitals to cope with infectious disease outbreaks (including those shown in Sidebar 3-7 on page 65). Hospitals are being alerted to deal with the following scenarios:

- How to manipulate the hospital's HVAC system to turn patient rooms into negative pressure air rooms and exhaust the infectious air to the outside without returning it to the building
- How to find products that can be affixed to walls or ceilings to convert normal patient rooms into negative pressure air rooms
- How to set up a temporary structure within a designated area of the community that would enable a certain segment of the population to be isolated

And a working group at Tampa General Hospital has submitted, to the Florida Hospital Association for review by and input from other hospitals throughout the state the following proposed guidelines for arresting or preventing a disease outbreak. The hope is eventually to enact these recommendations to regulate patient placement and movement in case of a disease outbreak. The facility will do the following:

1. Accommodate 10 beds
2. Provide negative air pressure in relation to surrounding areas; minimum of one one-hundredth (.01) of an inch
3. Provide a magnahelic gauge to ensure that pressure differentials are maintained
4. Monitor continuously for negative air pressure
5. Provide at least 12 air changes per hour of circulation (supply and exhaust)
6. Ensure that air is exhausted to the outdoors on the roof of the facility through monitored HEPA filters; no air from this facility will be circulated to other areas
7. Provide supply air that is conditioned for summer or winter
8. Provide automatic door closers to ensure that doors are closed
9. Provide anterooms with air supply to maintain positive air pressure
10. Provide medical gas (oxygen, vacuum, and medical air) at each bed
11. Provide an emergency power supply to critical medical equipment and air-circulation equipment
12. Provide hand-cleaning facilities and toilet facilities

Designing for Patient Flow

A newer addition to the Leadership standards requires hospital leadership to develop and implement plans to identify and mitigate issues, in a hospital, that can interfere with efficient movement of patients across the continuum of care within an organization. The Joint Commission implemented this new standard to prevent patient crowding, a problem that can lead to lapses in patient safety and the quality of care.

Standard LD.3.15
The leaders develop and implement plans to identify and mitigate impediments to efficient patient flow throughout the hospital.

Achieving a smooth flow of patients through a health care facility requires an appropriate matching of capacity and demand, efficient and effective work flow, and a care environment that optimizes patient outcomes and staff performance. How the actual facility is designed can have considerable impact—either positive or negative—on patient flow.

Before beginning design, team members should examine all processes critical to patient flow through the hospital system—from the time the patient arrives, through admitting, patient assessment and treatment, and discharge—and determine how design and layout can improve patient flow. In planning and design, some actions organizations can take include the following:

Design a fast-track area. Many organizations are separating out their ED into two areas: fast track and trauma. The fast-track section services patients who need limited and specific care, such as stitches and treatment for broken bones, minor cuts, and so forth. The trauma section services patients who require more intensive treatment, such as medical, obstetric, psychiatric, and cardiac care. Each section has its own waiting room. By physically separating these two types of patients through design, the organization can keep patients flowing more smoothly through the ED.

Increase inpatient bed capacity. Many times slowdowns in patient flow occur because no inpatient beds are available. Patients are held in the emergency room or intensive care unit (ICU) until a bed is available. As the ED or ICU fills, and the exiting patients have not left, a patient flow issue can arise. After an organization examines its patient flow processes, it may determine that more inpatient beds are necessary.

Convert existing space. Sometimes adding inpatient beds is not possible, and organizations must work with what they have. Some organizations have redesigned their ED to include a private holding area, where patients can safely wait until a bed becomes available. Such areas are made by converting space from other parts of the ED, including break rooms, waiting rooms, and hallways.[4] Other organizations design private rooms that can quickly convert to semiprivate rooms during increases in patient flow. By opening up more beds, the organization improves the flow.

Buy efficient equipment. Telemetry, radiology, and computer equipment can all slow down or streamline the patient care process, depending on the type of equipment. Organizations should consider using efficient technology that reduces diagnostic and treatment delays so patient flow can be enhanced.

Standardize room layout. As mentioned previously, standardizing patient room layouts can improve patient and staff safety. It can also improve efficiency because staff know where everything is located. This improvement in efficiency can enhance patient flow.

Maintaining Patient Flow During Construction

Renovation and construction must occur without interrupting the usual patient care provided by a health care organization. Through proactive space planning, an organization can renovate in phases to maintain patient flow. In Cabell Huntington Hospital (CHH), in Huntington, West Virginia, the in-house construction team preserved patient flow during construction by using adjacent space freed up by another department that was relocated. The team readied the adjacent space for patients and moved them into that space. Then the team built a number of ED rooms that functioned "as a pod," got the pod ready for patient care, and moved patients into the new pod. Pod by pod, work progressed quickly during a six-month period and was completed two months ahead of schedule. "We never dropped below the number of rooms we had before, but when we were done, we had five additional ED treatment rooms and three additional immediate care rooms," says Paul Lageman, R.N., director of emergency services at CHH.[5]

Designing for Security

Joint Commission Standard EC.2.10 requires organizations to address their security risks. Organizations constructing or renovating facilities must keep security issues in mind during planning and design. This could include choosing appropriate alarm systems, door locks, keyless entry systems, closed-circuit televisions, metal detectors, panic buttons, and so forth. It could also mean designing floor layouts to preserve the safety and security of staff and patients.

Standard EC.2.10
(AHC, BHC, CAH, HAP, LAB, LTC, OBS, OME)
The organization identifies and manages its security risks.

If the organization is building an ED, security issues are particularly important. The ED is an area of a health care organization that is ripe for violence. Care recipients arrive in acute physical or psychological stress, yet the nature of emergency medicine demands fast-paced assessment, treatment, and disposition of the care recipient. To minimize the potential for violent behavior, health care organizations need to design EDs that tightly control access to each of the four major ED areas: waiting, triage, treatment, and seclusion.

Waiting Area

As a reception area for ambulatory care recipients and a general waiting area, this part of the ED can accommodate relatively free access. In smaller facilities that have minimal staff, organizations may want to design the entry to be locked but able to be readily opened for arrivals. This could include the use of a night bell, remote unlocking, and voice communication devices. Even in larger facilities, where the entry point is open 24 hours per day, locking hardware will make it possible, should circumstances warrant, to quickly impose a total lockdown of the ED.

The admissions function usually occupies space in the waiting area, and an admissions clerk is often the first person approached when the triage area or signs pointing to it are not readily apparent. To protect the admissions clerk from being grabbed or struck, a facility can enclose or semi-enclose the desk area; if this area does not open directly to the treatment area, it should be locked.

Triage Area

The triage area should be configured in much the same manner as the admissions desk area, with the exception that a care recipient must be able to easily access the triage area. A direct opening from triage to the treatment area should be available.

Treatment Area

Approximately half of all violent acts that occur in the ED take place in the treatment area. Good security practice dictates that all entry points to this area be locked, including those to the waiting room, x-ray, and laboratories. Either card access or push button locks can allow for staff entry.

Seclusion Room

Large EDs usually have dedicated seclusion rooms; smaller EDs often have rooms that can quickly be converted to this purpose. A seclusion room must allow for unhindered observation of care recipients. Because it will be free of any equipment and designed for care recipient safety, it may also be used as a police prisoner holding area.

Designing for Life Safety

The Joint Commission, through Standard EC.5.20, requires all facilities, whether newly constructed, renovated, or existing, to comply with the *Life Safety Code®* *(LSC)*.* Developed by the National Fire Protection Agency (NFPA), this code helps organizations protect patients, staff, and visitors from threats posed by fire.

There are two ways in which organizations must comply with the *LSC* during the building process. When organizations plan and design a building, they must ensure that the building meets the requirements outlined by the *LSC*. In addition, organizations must ensure that compliance is maintained during the construction process. Ensuring *LSC* compliance in design is discussed in this section. (For information on complying with the *LSC* during construction, *see* page 107.)

Standard EC.5.20

(AHC, BHC, CAH, HAP, LAB, LTC, OBS, OME, HDS)
Newly constructed and existing environments are designed and maintained to comply with the LSC. (CAH: Corresponds to COP 485.623(d)(1), (d)(2), (d)(3), and (d)(5)(i-ii))

Defend in Place

A significant requirement of the *LSC* is ensuring that a building allows for a "defend in place" response to a fire. In a health care building where patients are incapacitated, the *LSC* requires that occupants be protected without evacuation. This concept is called defend in place, and the design of the health care facility plays a critical role in ensuring this.

The *LSC* outlines five levels of defense (*see* Figures 3-5 to 3-9 on pages 70–72):

1. *The room.* Closing the corridor door should provide the initial protection.
2. *The smoke compartment.* A patient care unit with 30 or more patients sleeping overnight requires two smoke compartments, both limited to 22,500 square feet. The smoke compartments may be less, and do not need to be equally sized.
3. *The floor assembly.* All shafts, chutes, and penetrations must be constructed and protected in a manner to create an adequate building separation for the occupants floor to floor. This separation may be by fire dampers at the floor location, or by creating a protected vertical shaft.
4. *Building components, such as fire-rated doors, smoke barriers, fire alarms, and smoke detectors.* Smoke barriers must be continuous from outside wall to outside wall, from one smoke barrier to another, or a combination thereof. They must be continuous through all concealed spaces, including those found above a ceiling. Any penetrations of the smoke barrier, by duct work, pipes, cables, conduits, and so forth, must be protected by approved smoke dampers that close on activation of smoke detectors, unless it is a fully ducted system and an approved automatic sprinkler system is on either side of the smoke barrier.
5. *Exits to the outside.* After occupants are outside they should be on a sidewalk or solid surface that allows for safe exiting.

For health care organizations that provide outpatient services, such as ambulatory care facilities, the *LSC* does not require defend-in-place strategies; however, it does require prompt evacuation. For residential facilities, such as dormitories or lodgings, the *LSC* requires alarms and evacuation.

In addition to defend in place, the *LSC* addresses the size, features, layout, and safety precautions associated with many other aspects of building design and layout, including, but not limited to, the following:

- Corridors
- Rooms
- Doors
- Vertical openings, such as elevators, escalators, and linen and waste chutes

---

*Life Safety Code® is a registered trademark of the National Fire Protection Association (NFPA, Quincy, MA.

- Exits
- Sprinkler systems
- Utilities

The scope of this publication does not allow an in-depth discussion of the *LSC* requirements. For specific information, organizations should obtain a copy of the requirements and consider how they apply to the building project.

Designing for Infection Control

As with designing for life safety, there are multiple opportunities to protect patients from infection simply through thoughtful facility design. During the planning and design phases, organizations have the opportunity to design layouts and include equipment that helps prevent the spread of infection.

Following are some things organizations should consider when designing for infection control:

Number and placement of hand sinks. Studies have shown that frequently placed hand-washing sinks can help encourage staff compliance with hand hygiene protocols.

Number and placement of alcohol-based hand rub dispensers. To make hand hygiene more convenient, organizations should consider having such a dispenser in every patient room. Some individuals have expressed concern that alcohol-based hand rubs are flammable. Although acknowledging this concern, the Joint Commission believes, based on NFPA studies, that the typical alcohol gel and foam dispensers in the health care setting are of such limited size and volume that the alcohol gel's contribution to the hazard of acceleration of fire development or fire spread is "negligible."

Number and placement of negative pressure rooms. These types of rooms can keep infected air from seeping out into other areas of the facility. Such rooms are appropriate for patient isolation areas, decontamination rooms, and cleanrooms. Depending on the size and scope of the facility and the building project, several of these rooms may be necessary. The location of showers, tubs, and restrooms in relation to the negative pressure rooms is also an important issue to consider.

Effective engineering of the HVAC system. An effective HVAC system can reduce the spread of infection. Conversely a poorly designed system can enhance the likelihood that cross contamination will occur. Effective HVAC systems may include multiple HEPA filtration units to help minimize particles in high-risk areas, such as the operating room (OR) and isolation rooms. HVAC systems should be able to adequately maintain the appropriate humidity, temperature, and air exchanges to address the needs of each area of the facility. Consideration regarding where to place AHUs, controls, and alarms must also be reviewed. Contingency plans should be made during power outages for rooms on normal power.

Effective water systems. Water, if not kept at the right temperature and pH, can breed mold or other contaminants, which can cause problems in some patients. Some organizations use chlorination to ensure the proper pH, while others use a copper-silver ionization process. In the latter system, the proper combination of copper and silver in the water breaks down biofilm.

Minimizing the use of carpeting. Carpeting can be harder to maintain than some other floor finishes. Organizations should consider eliminating the use of carpeting in areas at high risk for the spread of infection, such as patient rooms, surgical areas, and so forth, because the cleaning process itself might aerosolize fungal spores.

"Carpets in health care facilities should always have impermeable backing, chemically welded seams, and antistatic properties," says Jean Young, A.S.I.D., Young + Company, San Diego. Young said some of the newer carpeting materials are very thin rather than plushy and have vinyl backing, so liquids stay right on top and can be squeegeed out; like vinyl, they show puddles clearly.[6] If an organization does choose to use carpeting, it must consider how well the carpeting will stand up to frequent cleaning and decontamination. Carpets should be vacuumed daily and periodically steam cleaned. Organizations should consider how much it will cost to maintain the carpet and what to do with patients while carpets are being decontaminated.

Selecting appropriate wall sealants. Although the evidence suggests that walls and ceilings are not a major source for health care–associated infection, wall coverings should be fluid resistant and easily cleaned, especially in areas where contact with blood or body fluids may occur (for example, laboratories and operating rooms). Organizations should consider using epoxy paint when sealing the walls of such high-risk areas. This can prevent the spread of mold into high-risk areas. Northwestern Memorial Hospital used epoxy paint in its new building to seal operating rooms. When a leaking flash sterilizer, which had already saturated two entire walls in a surgical suite, finally burst and flooded an OR, the epoxy paint was the only thing between the mold and the patient. There was a lot of mold, but not one patient was

FIGURE 3-5. **Defend in Place—Level 1: Room**

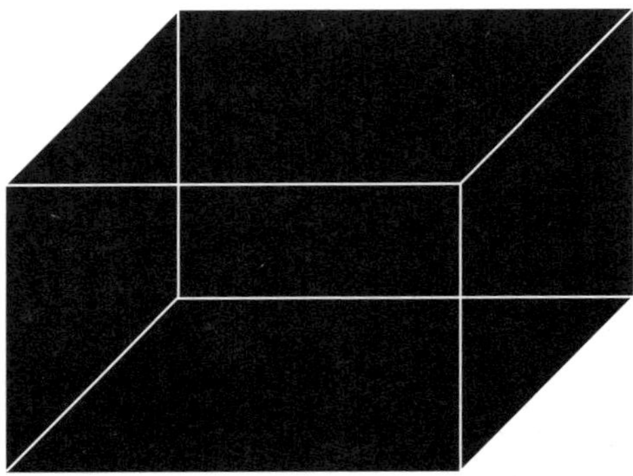

The first level of defense is the room. Closing the corridor door provides initial protection to the occupants.

In a patient care unit, there is no requirement in the *Life Safety Code*® for patient room separation above the ceiling (sound and other issues may supersede this, however).

Occupants in a room with a fire leave the room to the safety of the corridor, which is why door closing is so important.

FIGURE 3-6. **Defend in Place—Level 2: Smoke Compartment**

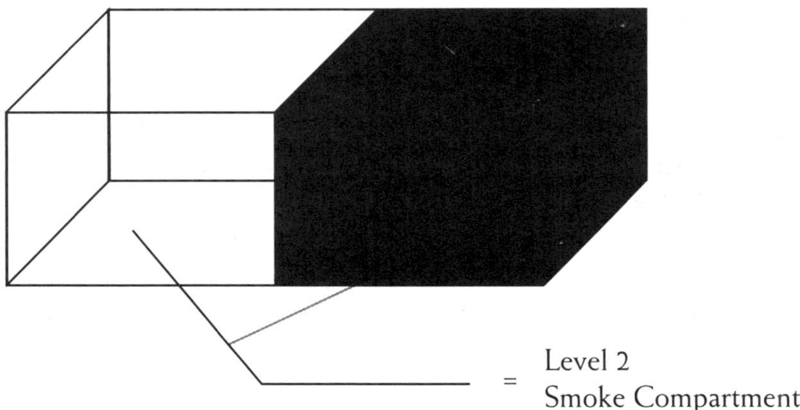

After the room, this is the second unit of defense.

As we will discover later, a patient care unit with 30 or more patients sleeping overnight requires two smoke compartments, both limited to 22,500 square feet. The smoke compartments may be less, and do not need to be equally sized.

FIGURE 3-7. Defend in Place—Level 3: Floor Assembly

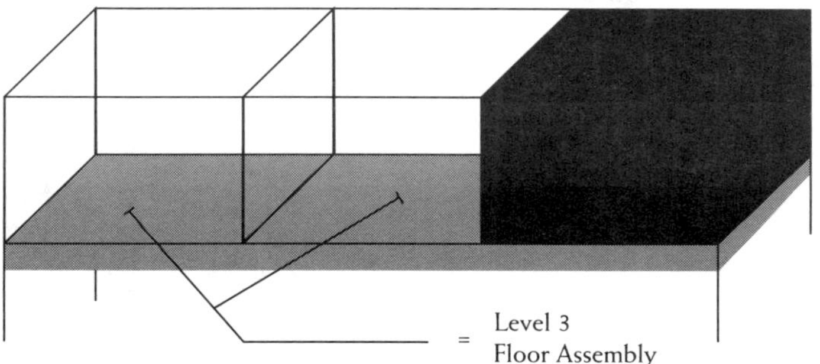

Separating the occupants by at least 2-hour construction, the floor assembly is the 3rd unit of defense.

All shafts, chutes, and penetrations must be constructed and protected in a manner to create an adequate building separation for the occupants floor to floor. This separation may be by fire dampers at the floor location, or

Creating a protected vertical shaft:

If < 3stories, existing construction, separate from the rest of the occupancy with ½-hour construction.
NOTE: 1-hour new construction.

If > 4 stories, 2-hour construction (existing and new construction).

FIGURE 3-8. Defend in Place—Level 4: Building Components

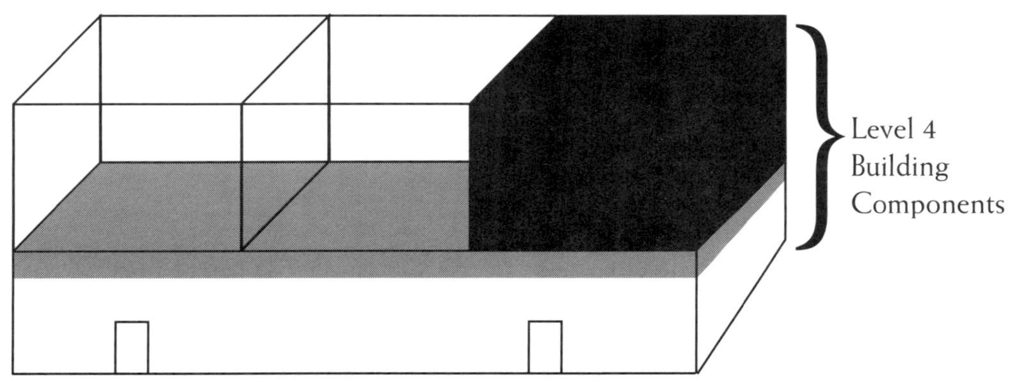

Building components, such as fire-rated doors, smoke barriers, features of fire safety (fire alarm, smoke detection, etc.) all contribute to the 4th unit of defense for the building occupants.

FIGURE 3-9. Defend in Place—Level 5: Exits

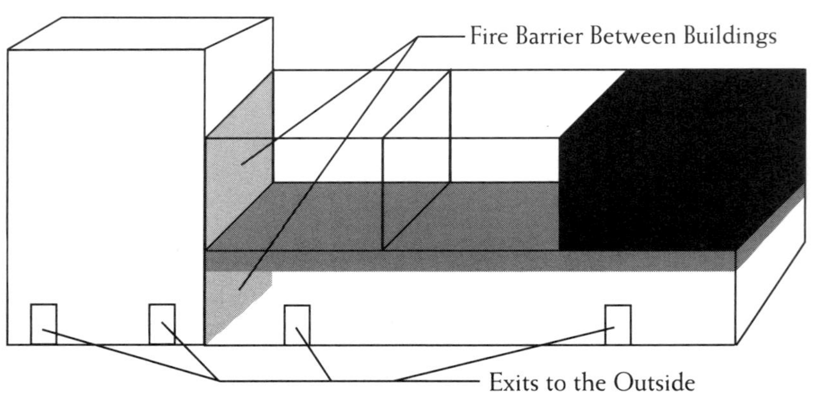

The 5th unit of defense is the exits to the outside. Ultimately, leaving the building provides the highest level of safety.

Horizontal exits (such as the plane between the buildings) creates an equivalent level of defense as the exits to the outside. These assemblies begin at the lowest level and extend to the roof deck. Construction is at least 2-hour, and all penetrations are protected with a 2-hour fire-resistant-rated assembly. When the occupant passes through the horizontal exit, he or she has essentially changed occupancies. The integrity of the horizontal exit is the same as a stair tower construction. (LSC 101-2000, 7.2.4 and 18 / 19.2.2.5)

When the occupants leave the building, they should find themselves on the way to a public access. This should be obvious and substantial (i.e., a sidewalk or solid surface to allow occupants to safely exit the building).

Fire Safety Planning would expect occupants to gather at a predetermined location to account for all occupants (review fire plans and ask staff).

harmed because the epoxy paint held.[7]

Selecting appropriate finishes. Plastic holds germs longer than stainless steel, so organizations should try to use stainless steel if at all possible. Finishings around plumbing fixtures should be smooth and water resistant. In addition, pipe penetrations and joints should be tightly sealed.

Appropriate ceiling design. Acoustical tiles should be avoided in high-risk areas because they might support microbial growth when wet. False ceilings, which can harbor dust and pests, should be avoided in high-risk areas unless adequately sealed.

Considering infection control in the laboratory. Such considerations should include the appropriate number of negative pressure areas, hoods, and the proper placement of hand-washing sinks. More on this topic can be found in Appendix A.

Considering infection control in the pharmacy. Such considerations should include complying with USP 797 and NIOSH guidelines. More on this topic can be found in Appendix B.

Like safety, designing for IC requires the design team to look at the layout in design through an IC perspective. Involving IC professionals early on in the planning process can ensure that IC issues are addressed.

Case Study 3-5. Expansion Provides Golden Opportunity

St. Rita's Medical Center Keeps Environment of Care Issues Front and Center in Planning Process

A major hospital expansion project can be a golden opportunity to create a superior environment of care (EC). Lack of focus during planning, however, can lead to EC problems that persist for years. For St. Rita's Medical Center in Lima, Ohio, which recently broke ground on a $130 million expansion, EC issues were at the heart of the planning process from the very beginning.

Set the Tone Up Front

St. Rita's Medical Center is a 424-bed hospital that provides acute care and other health services to residents of west central Ohio. During the past several years, the center has experienced a surge in patient volume. "We have been up against bed capacity issues for some time," says Brian Smith, chief operating officer and executive vice president of St. Rita's. "We are already over 80% in key areas and 90% in others."

In 2001 the organization addressed the issue head-on by initiating a fully scoped master facility planning process. One of the first steps was to bring in an actuarial firm to project local health care demand. "The data showed a bed shortfall in less than 10 years," Smith says. By the second half of 2002, the medical center had engaged a leading health care architectural firm and the planning process was well under way. In March of 2005, construction began on a 270,000-square-foot expansion that will increase bed capacity by nearly 20%. The doors are scheduled to open in 2007.

According to Smith, the biggest lesson from the hospital's planning experience is the importance of creating a sense of priority for EC issues: "We set the tone up front so that life safety and infrastructure got as much discussion and energy as any other part of the project."

Planning for a Secure Environment

Smith said one key to incorporating EC safety and security standards in the planning process was involving stakeholders from the community.

To enhance life safety planning, project leaders invited the local fire chief to take an active part in the design process. "We asked for his input on how facility designs could impact the department's ability to respond to an emergency," states Smith. The chief red-flagged a large entrance canopy that could have posed access problems for fire trucks. He also pointed out landscaping elements that could potentially impede rescue workers. "In our own little world, we would not have caught these kinds of things," Smith says. "Putting life safety on an equal footing in the planning process allowed this dialogue to take place."

Planners also sought input on security issues. "The campus police chief was involved in key project committees and attended the weekly construction meeting," Smith stated. The local chief of police also took part in discussions. Their input helped the project team enhance ED security by creating entrances and exits that control patient traffic. Patient flow was also a central issue in emergency management—designs now ensure the ability to lock down the ED and move patients through without assigning temporary rooms.

The planning team gave careful attention to the problem of bottlenecking in general. Blueprints call for a new Outpatient Services Department just off the main lobby that will give patients quick access to preadmission testing, diagnostics, and lab work. In addition, Smith says, the team incorporated hazardous materials management into overall materials management planning: "Our new loading dock will include an area that we can use to manage short-term storage of hazardous materials."

Upgrading Infrastructure

Smith notes that the planning team took a long-term approach to infrastructure issues. The result: business-oriented decisions with a positive impact on EC compliance.

The hospital's utilities plan focuses on a new electrical substation and a new boiler. Smith says the new energy center will have the capacity to support EC needs well into the future. "We built in additional redundancy to handle further growth for the next 25 years," he says. The new energy

Continued on page 74

Continued from page 73

center is also a major part of the hospital's emergency power plan.

From the beginning, states Smith, the planning team tried to take into account the impact of upcoming technology on infrastructure needs. As a result, the new facility will include infrastructure to support wireless communication and computerized prescriber order entry. The team also examined the issue of medical equipment management, creating back hallways that will allow staff to move equipment throughout the hospital quickly and with minimal disruption to the patient environment.

Although not exclusively part of the expansion project, the medical center's risk-assessment program contributed significantly to the planning process. According to Smith, the program identified the following risk areas that are being addressed in the expansion design:

- Pediatrics—new traffic flow layout will reduce the risk of infant abduction
- Laboratory—new design will head off potential problems with egress standards
- Nutrition services—new kitchen takes into account trends in worker's comp

Putting Patients First

"One of our basic design standards was that the patient has to come first," says Smith. "Everything has to be done with an eye toward patient safety." Special committees examined the patient experience (both inpatient and outpatient) and provided input on the design of the physical EC.

Addressing the issue of space, the planning team designed a new 390-square-foot universal patient room. "We took into account the family presence," Smith states. "There is a distinct zone for family members and a distinct zone for caregivers." New anterooms, he noted, will help triple isolation capacity.

Another core issue was light. "One of our commitments," says Smith, "was that at least 70% of patient areas have access to natural light." He believes this decision will positively impact both energy usage and patient outcomes.

Air quality also figured prominently in the planning process. One of the main features of the facility design is a new HVAC system. In addition, project leaders have been careful to guard air quality during construction. Work crews and hospital staff follow positive pressure and air return protocols, maintain fire-retardant plastic barriers, and measure air quality every four hours. "We follow the highest standards," Smith says. He noted that IC staff is involved in weekly construction meetings and conduct weekly rounds of the work sites.

Key Factors and Top Strategies

According to Smith, two factors helped St. Rita's Medical Center keep EC issues "front and center" during the expansion planning process.

One was getting leadership involved from the very beginning. "By involving the steering committee in the master planning process," he says, "everyone came to the next step of the journey fully informed." He notes that an earlier attempt at facility planning failed because "it happened in a small back room."

The second factor? "You need a facilities person who truly thinks with a business mind, someone who can speak the language of operations and capital folks." Smith says that Director of Facilities Ron Connovich, who showed a strong ability to make the business case for EC enhancements, was a major asset to the St. Rita's project.

With the design phase of the St. Rita's expansion complete, Smith offers the following strategies for a successful facility planning process:

1. Involve clinicians. Success depends on operational, facilities, and clinical leaders working together. "All three need to be at the table."
2. Partner with professionals who are experienced in health care. Architectural, engineering, and construction management firms should have specific hospital experience—plus health care engineering credentials.
3. Do your homework up front. "Understand your demand and your needs—define the problem and then define the solution."

Case-at-a-Glance on next page

CASE AT A GLANCE

■ **Main challenge**
To create design options for a surge facility. Maintain focus on EC issues during the planning process for a major hospital expansion project.

■ **Issues**
Address patient capacity and patient flow concerns while standardizing infrastructure throughout several components of a large hospital facility.

■ **Joint Commission Standards**
All EC standards, especially: EC.1.10: The hospital manages safety risks. EC.5.20, Newly constructed and existing environments of care are designed and maintained to comply with the *Life Safety Code®*. EC.8.10: The hospital establishes and maintains an appropriate environment. EC.8.30: The hospital manages the design and building of the environment when it is renovated, altered, or newly created.

■ **Solutions**
Involve all stakeholders—organizational, clinical, and facilities leaders, plus local safety officials—in the planning process. Make the business case for focusing on EC needs. In all decisions, put the patient first.

■ **Outcome**
A master health care facility plan that incorporates the full range of safety, security, infrastructure, and healing environment EC standards.

Proactive Risk Assessment

Debris chutes extend from third-floor windows to dumpsters below. Cranes lift immense loads of gypsum board sheets up to the roof. Signs direct construction workers to the appropriate facility entrance. These are common sights around health care facilities nationwide as organizations refurbish or replace aging buildings to increase available capacity.

Construction or renovation in occupied health care facilities can result in environmental problems that compromise patient safety, such as the creation or spread of contaminants, noises, vibration, or disruption of essential services. For example, infections associated with the dispersal of airborne or waterborne microorganisms during construction have been linked to such factors as new fireproofing insulation, carpeting, ventilation system humidifiers, and many other items in the care environment.[8] In one construction project, demolition of a nearby wall would have caused harmful vibration to an adjoining neonatal intensive care unit.

The Joint Commission requires organizations to manage safety during the construction process. Standard EC.8.30 requires organizations to conduct a proactive risk assessment as part of the planning phase of new building construction or renovation. This proactive risk assessment should identify hazards that could potentially compromise patient care in occupied areas of the organization's buildings. The scope and nature of the construction activities will determine the extent of the risk assessment. The criteria used to assess risk should address the impact the construction will have on the following areas:

- Air quality
- Infection control
- Utility requirements or interruptions
- Noise
- Vibration
- Emergency procedures

A variety of ways to conduct a proactive risk assessment are available, and the Joint Commission does not specify how organizations should do it. The following paragraphs outline one approach to the assessment process.

Determine the Scope of the Assessment

A first step in the proactive risk assessment process is to identify the type of construction activity, ranging from minor work that doesn't generate dust to major demolition and construction that generates dust or debris and creates noise and vibration over a longer period. The type of construction will determine the scope of the assessment and what areas should be addressed. One note of caution: Just because a project is small doesn't mean there aren't significant risks that should be assessed. Often, it is the small projects that result in the most complication, because organizations overlook the risks involved. For example, a simple cabling project may require drilling through fire walls, interrupting utilities, or generating significant noise. Organizations should identify these risks in the proactive risk assessment process, just as they would identify larger-scale risks for a building addition.[9]

Select a Team

The proactive risk assessment is most effective when undertaken as a multidisciplinary team effort. Organizations may want to include people with expertise in IC, risk management, facility design, ventilation, safety, and epidemiology on the team. Certainly other members may be added as appropriate for the given situation. These may include building engineers and direct care supervisors. The contractor is another important member of the assessment team. He or she can bring experience from other organizations' building projects to the table and notice issues that health care organization staff may overlook.

Although all health care organization team members are important, the IC representative plays a special role on the proactive risk assessment team. This individual brings an understanding of the affected patient population, can assist with educating the construction workers on IC concerns, and provides other specific expertise.

The Association for Professionals in Infection Control and Epidemiology (APIC) recommends that after the risk assessment team is selected, an authority should be assigned to coordinate the process. It notes that contractor accountability for attention to IC issues should be written into the contract documents (*see* Chapter Four). Furthermore, APIC reminds organizations to focus not only on patients, but also on the risks to health care workers, volunteers, and the contractors themselves.

SIDEBAR 3-8.
Proactive Risk Assessment and ICRA

The terms proactive risk assessment and ICRA are often used interchangeably. In fact, the Joint Commission's requirement for the preconstruction risk assessment is essentially the same as the AIA's description of the ICRA. The only point of clarification is that the Joint Commission does not require that any one particular form be used to conduct this risk assessment. Some popular forms, one example of which is shown on pages 81–85, are only one way to satisfy the Joint Commission's requirement for conducting a preconstruction risk assessment. (It should also be noted that this form does not include assessments for noise and vibration, which both the Joint Commission and the AIA do require.)

Review Joint Commission, AIA, and CDC Guidelines

The Joint Commission is not the only organization that requires an assessment of constructions risks. The *American Institute of Architects (AIA) Guidelines* also require organizations to consider these risks. The guidelines state that "during the programming phase of a construction project, the owner shall provide an Infection Control Risk Assessment (ICRA)" to determine the potential risk of transmission of various agents in the facility. An ICRA is not only conducted before construction begins, but should be a continuous process starting during planning and continuing throughout design and construction. An ICRA should be conducted by a panel with expertise in IC, risk management, facility design, construction ventilation, safety, and epidemiology. According to the AIA, the panel should provide updated documentation of the risk assessment through planning, design, and construction. The ICRA should only address building areas anticipated to be affected by construction.[10] Construction issues to assess in the ICRA may include, but are not limited to, the following:

- Disruption of essential services
- Relocation or placement of patients
- Barrier placements to control airborne contaminants
- Debris cleanup and removal
- Traffic flow

The concept of a proactive risk assessment is also supported by the CDC's Draft Guidelines for Environmental Infection Control in Healthcare Facilities, 2001 edition, which suggests three major considerations:

1. The design and function of the new area
2. The risk of airborne disease transmission
3. Preventive measures to contain dust and moisture

The CDC also suggests giving consideration to construction projects that occur outside the health care facility's walls and perhaps even outside the property lines. Adjacent construction, whether undertaken by the health care facility or others, can affect patients within the facility if dust and airborne contaminants are permitted to enter the building via air intakes or other openings.

Create a Matrix

Many organizations construct a matrix to ensure the proper consideration of the risks involved in a construction project, the patients affected by the project, and the appropriate responses for the risks and patients involved. The matrix should include four types of information:

1. The types of patients affected
2. The nature of the project
3. The types of issues involved with the project
4. Actions to minimize risks

The Type of Patients Affected. If the construction project involves areas where immunocompromised patients are being treated, the risks of construction will be higher than in office spaces. Organizations should differentiate between low-, medium-, and high-risk areas.

The Nature of the Project. As previously mentioned, the nature of the construction project can influence the amount of risk involved.

The Types of Issues Involved with the Project. These can vary depending on the type of project. Some common risks include the following:

- *Dust and fumes.* These can compromise patient safety, even in small-scale projects. Dust can have severe effects on asthmatic patients. Volatile organic compounds, which are chemicals typically contained in cleaners, paint, adhesives, and the off-gas of new carpeting and upholstered furniture, can cause adverse health effects.
- *Mold.* Mold occurs on a construction site when materials get wet. This could be due to a burst pipe, water leak, or rain intrusion. These scenarios are common to most construction projects. Mold can be hazardous to patients with compromised immune systems and others. The CDC offers specific guidelines on how to handle materials that come in contact with moisture. Organizations must dry the materials completely before use or remove them within 72 hours. Some organizations choose to use a conservative approach to mold prevention and ban the use of materials that have become wet in construction projects.
- *Fungi.* When renovating an older building, construction teams have to deal with fungi, such as *Aspergillus.* Sources of fungi include outdoor air; previously water-damaged ceilings, plaster, or drywall; construction dust; excavation; wet areas in the HVAC system; living plants; and bird and bat droppings. Fungal spores very easily become airborne after being disturbed, and handlers must take care to carefully wet any affected material before its removal so that spores do not become airborne. Construction is associated as a risk factor for opportunistic airborne fungal infection in immunocompromised patients because normal ventilation may be disrupted, possibly releasing hazardous airborne spores into the environment. The phases of construction that usually create the greatest risk include demolition, window or wall removal, ventilation and utility outages, application of volatile chemicals, and placement of combustion engines.
- *Hazardous material.* A renovation process can sometimes disturb existing materials, and some of these materials could be hazardous to the health of patients. For example, asbestos and lead paint are still present in some facilities, and they have well-documented health risks to all populations. Mercury was commonly used in earlier decades for temperature gauges and switches, which can still be found in research laboratories and health care facilities. Fluorescent lamps also have mercury in them. During construction, these instruments can break, releasing the highly toxic substance.
- *Water contaminants.* During construction projects, bacteria can enter the water system, thus contaminating it. Such bacteria could include *Legionella.*
- *Noise and vibration.* As previously mentioned, noise can have a detrimental effect on patient care, and vibration can affect delicate surgical procedures. Organizations should be aware of the impact of construction noise on patients and staff and work to minimize that impact when possible.
- *Emergency procedures.* Construction projects can dramatically impact an organization's emergency response procedures. Many times entrance and exits are moved, traffic is rerouted, and alarm systems are disabled. Organizations must consider how the facility would respond to an emergency during construction, including how the organization would defend in place and, if necessary, evacuate.
- *Utilities disruption.* During the course of construction, the organization may be required to shut off main power, heat, water, or air-conditioning. Organizations must consider the impact of these shutdowns on a system and patient level. For example, if the water is shut off for two hours, how will patients be affected? how will staff be affected? how will equipment be affected? What is the most appropriate time for the shutdown that will have the least impact?

Actions to Minimize Risks. These could include the following:

- *Project isolation.* Construction projects should be isolated from the rest of the facility. Large-scale projects, such as constructing a new wing or renovating an old one, might be easier to isolate than small-scale projects, such as painting a few rooms or repairing ceiling tiles. NFPA requires a two-hour separation from slab to slab to separate any construction areas from the rest of the building.
- *Work methods.* Organizations should consider all types of work methods that could reduce the likelihood of future patient safety problems. Using HEPA–filtered fan units and vacuums to minimize dust, working off hours or on weekends to reduce patient and staff impact, wetting down materials with a fine spray to prevent the spread of dust and

fungi, as appropriate, and other strategies could address risks.

• *An effective HVAC system.* Because virtually all buildings have some degree of recirculation in their ventilation systems, requiring both a supply and a return, careful proactive planning prevents buildingwide contamination during construction. This could include contamination from dust, fumes, or other airborne particles. To prevent contamination from the construction site, air must flow from clean to dirty. The facility's HVAC engineer must determine how to isolate the system. This may include sealing vents, adding additional filters, or using other means. Elevator shafts require special consideration because of their tendency to function like a chimney, drawing odors, dust, and fumes up through the shaft onto other floors. (*See* Sidebar 3-9 on page 79 for further ways to maintain indoor air quality.)

• *Negative pressure areas.* No matter how well an area is sealed with plastic sheeting or rigid barrier walls, air leaks can occur. Using negative pressure can prevent seepage into adjacent areas and can draw air containing dust, fumes, and other particles back into the construction area. Recirculation of air is prevented. Exhaust from the construction area should be filtered and directed outside to a predetermined area. Negative air machines, capable of drawing in and filtering up to 2,000 cubic feet of air per minute, can be used. Although these units used to be expensive, their cost has dropped and they work extremely well. HEPA–filtered units are capable of filtering out 99.97% of particulate matter. One down side to negative pressure machines is that they can be noisy. Organizations will need to address this noise during the proactive risk assessment process. Organizations should also assess how much negative pressure will be needed at the construction site, where the exhaust will go, how the pressure will be monitored, and whether to use existing equipment.[11] Negative pressure can also be used with small-scale projects. For example, if workers need to run wires above a ceiling, they can "contain" just the area they're working in by building a plastic cube around the work area and putting the cube under negative pressure with a small negative air unit or a HEPA–filtered vacuum cleaner. With proper exhausting outside the cube, dust and fumes can be kept from migrating to occupied areas.

• *Clean and dirty anterooms.* Just outside the construction site, organizations may wish to set up clean and dirty rooms. This will help construction workers remove particles, such as dust, fungi, and bacteria, from their person before leaving the project area. This can minimize the transfer of particles outside the construction zone.

• *Tacky mats.* By placing these at the entrance to and exit from the construction site, organizations can minimize the spread of dust and debris throughout the facility.

• *Covered containers for waste removal.* This can prevent the spread of odors, dust, and other particles that can cause patient harm. It also reduces volatile organic compounds (VOCs). Waste should be removed every day. In addition, containers of paints and adhesives should be kept closed when not in use.

• *Low-emitting materials.* As previously mentioned, by using low-emitting materials during construction, organizations can prevent off-gassing of VOCs and carcinogens into the air. This can preserve the environment as well as the safety of construction staff, health care organization staff, patients, and visitors.

• *Traffic control.* Preconstruction planning defines how workers will enter and exit the building and the route they'll take to the construction area. Separation of patient/visitor/staff traffic from construction traffic is highly desirable, if possible. Signs should direct patients, staff, and visitors away from the construction area.[8]

In larger buildings, it might be appropriate to designate freight elevators for construction traffic. These are designed for heavier use and are rarely used by patients. If this is not feasible, one or more elevator(s) can be "keyed off," allowing only construction staff use. Organizations should consider how to protect nonfreight elevators because they can be damaged quickly during construction. Placement of the construction office for large projects requires planning as well. An office trailer should not get in the way of entering or exiting patients, visitors, and staff.

• *Air and water testing.* While not required, organizations should consider frequently testing the air and water for contaminants during construction. Such contaminants could include *Aspergillus,* mold, dust, *Legionella, Pencillium,* and other infection-causing agents.

• *Monitoring immunocompromised patients for airborne infections during construction.*

• *Providing protective clothing for workers at the construction site.* This may be a coverall or other type of clothing.

• *Barriers.* Barriers can seal off the construction site. As part of the risk assessment, organizations should determine where to place barriers, with what materials to make barriers, and the life safety considerations associated with those barriers.[11]

• *Cleaning.* This could include wiping down work services with disinfectant, daily vacuuming with HEPA–filtered vacuums, or ensuring that all trash is removed from the construction site on a regular basis.

SIDEBAR 3-9. Air Quality Management During Construction

A comprehensive indoor air quality (IAQ) management plan incorporates strategies and technologies to control pollutant sources and interrupt contamination pathways. The following requirements are part of the draft "Green Guidelines for Healthcare Construction":

- In occupied buildings, seal the construction site with deck-to-deck partitions, with a two-hour fire-rated resistance, and maintain the construction area under negative pressure throughout the entire construction process.
- During construction meet or exceed the recommended Design Approaches of the Sheet Metal and Air Conditioning National Contractors Association (SMACNA) *IAQ Guideline for Occupied Buildings Under Construction,* 1995, Chapter 3.
- Manage the site in conjunction with the ICRA procedures outlined by the owner and designer. Meet or exceed the requirements outlined in SMACNA *IAQ Guideline for Occupied Buildings Under Construction,* 1995, Chapter 4.
- Protect absorptive materials from moisture damage while they are stored on site and after they are installed. Immediately remove from site and properly dispose of any materials with stains, mold, mildew, or other evidence of water damage and replace with new, undamaged materials.
- Schedule construction procedures to minimize exposure of absorbent materials to VOC emissions. For example, complete "wet" construction procedures such as painting and sealing before storing or installing "dry" absorbent materials such as carpet or ceiling tiles. These absorptive materials act as a "sink," retaining contaminants and releasing them over time.
- Seal ducts during transportation, delivery, and construction to prevent accumulation of construction dust and construction debris inside ducts.
- If air handlers must be used during construction, filtration media with a minimum efficiency report value (MERV) of 8 must be used at each return air grill, as determined by ASHRAE 52.2-1999.
- Replace all filtration media immediately prior to occupancy. Use filtration media with a MERV of 13, as determined by ASHRAE 52.2-1999 for media installed at the end of construction.
- For painting equipment, develop a plan requiring use of high-volume, low-pressure (HVLP) paint guns and implement the plan when painting equipment is used.

Documentation Requirements

- Prepare, implement, and maintain a written Construction IAQ Management Plan highlighting the SMACNA requirements.
- Compile technical data on filtration media, listing each air filter used during construction and at the end of construction. Include the MERV value, manufacturer name, and model number.
- Maintain a copy of the ICRA developed for the project, highlighting these and any additional measures used to minimize the impact of construction on adjacent areas.
- Prepare specifications requiring use of HVLP paint guns and certification by an authorized party that the plan was implemented, as applicable.

And either

- Document the five design approaches of SMACNA *IAQ Guideline for Occupied Buildings under Construction,* Chapter 3, which were used during building construction. Include a brief description of some of the important design approaches employed.

or

- Document the five management approaches of SMACNA *IAQ Guideline for Occupied Buildings Under Construction,* Chapter 4, which were used during building construction.

Reference Standards

- *Sheet Metal and Air Conditioning National Contractors Association (SMACNA) IAQ Guideline for Occupied Buildings Under Construction,* 2000.
- NIOSH Publication No. 99-113: *Control of Drywall Sanding Dust Exposures.*

Source: Green Guidelines for Healthcare Construction: Creating High Performance Healing Environments. Convened by the Center for Maximum Potential Building Systems. Sponsored by the American Society for Healthcare Engineering. Funding provided by the Merck Family Fund. Dec 2003 Version 1.0 PC; Draft for Public Comment. http://www.gghc.org.

Although organizations are free to conduct the proactive risk assessment in any way they see fit, some choose to use a matrix developed by Premier Safety Institute (*see* Figure 3-10 on pages 81–85). *Note: This form is often referred to as the ASHE ICRA document. It is an example of a form that organizations can adapt for use in their own facilities. While it is a useful tool, organizations should use the form as a source for creating their own matrix that specifically addresses the scope, needs, and characteristics of the particular organization. Simply using the tool "as is" may not provide the most targeted assessment. In addition, organizations should be aware that this particular form does NOT include assessments of utilities, noise, vibration, air flow, and emergency procedures. These are items that the Joint Commission does require as part of the proactive risk assessment.*

Implement the Assessment

When the proactive risk assessment is complete, it is up to the organization to implement appropriate recommendations to reduce and control the risks inherent in the project. Furthermore, the controls instituted as a result of the assessment must be enforced. Organizations should revisit the assessment throughout the construction process to ensure that all risks are being appropriately addressed.

It is essential that the proactive risk assessment process be documented. The organization is ultimately responsible for conducting the assessment and implementing recommendations. But responsibilities for specification and implementation also lie with the contractor on the project, and these responsibilities should be clearly outlined in the contract. For more information on the construction contract, see Chapter Four.

Standard EC.8.30

(AHC, BHC, CAH, HAP, LAB, LTC)

The organization manages the design and building of the environment when it is renovated, altered, or newly created.

Elements of Performance

1. *(AHC, BHC, CAH, HAP, LTC) When planning for the size, configuration, and equipping of the space of renovated, altered, or new construction, the hospital uses one of the following: applicable state rules and regulations;* Guidelines for Design and Construction of Hospitals and Health Care Facilities, *2001 edition, published by the AIA; or similar standards or guidelines that provide design criteria.*

2. *(AHC, BHC, CAH, HAP, LTC) When planning demolition, construction, or renovation, the organization conducts a proactive risk assessment using risk criteria to identify hazards that could potentially compromise care, treatment, and services in occupied areas of the organization's buildings. The scope and nature of the activities should determine the extent of risk assessment.*

3. *(AHC, BHC, CAH, HAP, LTC) When planning demolition, construction, or renovation, the organization uses risk criteria that address the impact of demolition, renovation, or new construction on air-quality requirements, infection control, utility requirements, noise, vibration, and emergency procedures.*

4. *(AHC, BHC, CAH, HAP, LTC) When planning demolition, construction, or renovation, the organization selects and implements proper controls, as required, to reduce risk and minimize impact of these activities.*

5. *(LAB) When planning for the size, configuration, and equipping of the space of renovated, altered, or new construction, the laboratory uses one of the following as applicable: applicable state rules and regulations; Laboratory Design guidelines published by the NCCLS;* Guidelines for Design and Construction of Hospitals and Health Care Facilities, *2001 edition, published by the AIA; or similar standards or guidelines that provide equivalent design criteria. (See Appendix A for more information on designing for laboratories.)*

6. *(LAB) When site conditions or specific clinical needs require deviation from the referenced guidelines or standards, the laboratory identifies, when appropriate, the need for specialized staff training to effectively use the space and equipment provided.*

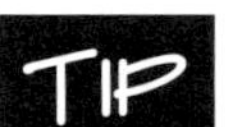

When scheduling a construction project, organizations must ensure that life safety is maintained. Project and facility managers should pay attention to the project schedule to ensure that risky situations aren't created. For example, fire alarms should not be taken offline at the same time as sprinklers. In addition, burn permits should not be released if the sprinklers and alarms are not working. Organizations should require that contractors coordinate work so that safety can be ensured.[12] ■

FIGURE 3-10. Sample ICRA Matrix of Precautions for Construction and Renovation

Step 1: Using the following table, identify the Type of Construction Project Activity (Type A–D)

TYPE A	**Inspection and noninvasive activities** Includes but is not limited to: • Removal of ceiling tiles for visual inspection (limited to 1 tile per 50 square feet) • Painting (but not sanding) • Wallcovering, electrical trim work, minor plumbing, and activities that do not generate dust or require cutting of walls or access to ceilings other than for visual inspection
TYPE B	**Small-scale, short-duration activities that create minimal dust** Includes but is not limited to: • Installation of telephone and computer cabling • Access to chase spaces • Cutting of walls or ceiling where dust migration can be controlled
TYPE C	**Work that generates a moderate to high level of dust or requires demolition or removal of any fixed building components or assemblies** Includes but is not limited to: • Sanding of walls for painting or wall covering • Removal of floor coverings, ceiling tiles, and casework • New wall construction • Minor duct work or electrical work above ceilings • Major cabling activities • Any activity that cannot be completed within a single work shift
TYPE D	**Major demolition and construction projects** Includes but is not limited to: • Activities that require consecutive work shifts • Requires heavy demolition or removal of a complete cabling system • New construction

Step 1: ______________________________

Step 2: Using the following table, identify the Patient Risk Groups that will be affected. If more than one risk group will be affected, select the higher-risk group:

Low Risk	**Medium Risk**	**High Risk**	**Highest Risk**
• Office areas	• Cardiology • Echocardiography • Endoscopy • Nuclear medicine • Physical therapy • Radiology/MRI • Respiratory therapy	• CCU • Emergency room • Labor and delivery • Laboratories (specimen) • Newborn nursery • Outpatient surgery • Pediatrics • Pharmacy • Postanesthesia care unit • Surgical units	• Any area caring for immunocompromised patients • Burn unit • Cardiac cath lab • Central sterile supply • Intensive care units • Medical unit • Negative pressure isolation rooms • Oncology • Operating rooms, including C-section rooms

Step 2: ______________________________

____

Continued on page 82

FIGURE 3-10. Sample ICRA Matrix of Precautions for Construction and Renovation, continued

Step 3: Match the Patient Risk Group (Low, Medium, High, Highest) with the planned…
Construction Project Type (A, B, C, D) on the following matrix, to find the…
Class of Precautions (I, II, III, or IV) or level of IC activities required.

Class I–IV or Color-Coded Precautions are delineated on the following page.

IC Matrix-Class of Precautions: Construction Project by Patient Risk

Construction Project Type

Patient Risk Group	TYPE A	TYPE B	TYPE C	TYPE D
LOW Risk Group	I	II	II	III/IV
MEDIUM Risk Group	I	II	III	IV
HIGH Risk Group	I	II	III/IV	IV
HIGHEST Risk Group	II	III/IV	III/IV	IV

Note: IC approval will be required when the Construction Activity and Risk Level indicate that **Class III** or **Class IV** control procedures are necessary.

Step 3: ______________________________

Description of Required IC Precautions by Class

	During Construction Project	Upon Completion of Project
CLASS I	1. Execute work by methods to minimize raising dust from construction operations. 2. Immediately replace a ceiling tile displaced for visual inspection.	1. Clean work area upon completion of task.
CLASS II	1. Provide active means to prevent airborne dust from dispersing into atmosphere. 2. Water mist work surfaces to control dust while cutting. 3. Seal unused doors with duct tape. 4. Block off and seal air vents. 5. Place dust mat at entrance and exit of work area. 6. Remove or isolate HVAC system in areas where work is being performed.	1. Wipe work surfaces with disinfectant. 2. Contain construction waste before transport in tightly covered containers. 3. Wet mop and/or vacuum with HEPA–filtered vacuum before leaving work area. 4. Remove isolation of HVAC system in areas where work is being performed.
CLASS III	1. Remove or isolate HVAC system in area where work is being done to prevent contamination of duct system. 2. Complete all critical barriers (that is, sheetrock, plywood, plastic) to seal area from nonwork area or implement control cube method (cart with plastic covering and sealed connection to work site with HEPA vacuum for vacuuming prior to exit) before construction begins. 3. Maintain negative air pressure within work site utilizing HEPA–equipped air filtration units. 4. Contain construction waste before transport in tightly covered containers. 5. Cover transport receptacles or carts. Tape covering unless solid lid.	1. Do not remove barriers from work area until completed project is inspected by the owner's safety department and IC department and thoroughly cleaned by the owner's environmental services department. 2. Remove barrier materials carefully to minimize spreading of dirt and debris associated with construction. 3. Vacuum work area with HEPA–filtered vacuums. 4. Wet mop area with disinfectant. 5. Remove isolation of HVAC system in areas where work is being performed.

Continued on page 83

FIGURE 3-10. Sample ICRA Matrix of Precautions for Construction and Renovation, continued

	During Construction Project	Upon Completion of Project
CLASS IV	1. Isolate HVAC system in area where work is being done to prevent contamination of duct system. 2. Complete all critical barriers (that is, sheetrock, plywood, plastic) to seal area from nonwork area or implement control cube method (cart with plastic covering and sealed connection to work site with HEPA vacuum for vacuuming prior to exit) before construction begins. 3. Maintain negative air pressure within work site utilizing HEPA–equipped air filtration units. 4. Seal holes, pipes, conduits, and punctures appropriately. 5. Construct anteroom and require all personnel to pass through this room so they can be vacuumed using a HEPA vacuum cleaner before leaving work site, or they can wear cloth or paper coveralls that are removed each time they leave the work site. 6. All personnel entering work site are required to wear shoe covers. Shoe covers must be changed each time the worker exits the work area. 7. Do not remove barriers from work area until completed project is inspected by the owner's safety department and IC department and thoroughly cleaned by the owner's environmental services department.	1. Remove barrier material carefully to minimize spreading of dirt and debris associated with construction. 2. Contain construction waste before transport in tightly covered containers. 3. Cover transport receptacles or carts. Tape covering unless solid lid. 4. Vacuum work area with HEPA–filtered vacuums. 5. Wet mop area with disinfectant. 6. Remove isolation of HVAC system in areas where work is being performed.

Step 4. Identify the areas surrounding the project area, assessing potential impact.

UNIT BELOW	UNIT ABOVE	LATERAL	LATERAL	BEHIND	FRONT
Risk Group	Risk Group	Risk Group	Risk Group	Risk Group	Risk Group

Step 5. Identify specific site of activity; for example, patient rooms, medication room, and so on.

Step 6. Identify issues related to ventilation, plumbing, and electrical in terms of the occurrence of probable outages.

Step 7. Identify containment measures, using prior assessment. What types of barriers? (For example, solid wall barriers.) Will HEPA filtration be required?
(Note: Renovation/construction area shall be isolated from the occupied areas during construction and shall be negative with respect to surrounding areas.)

Step 8. Consider potential risk of water damage. Is there a risk due to compromising structural integrity? (For example, wall, ceiling, roof.)

Step 9. Work hours: Can or will the work be done during nonpatient care hours?

Step 10. Do plans allow for adequate number of isolation or negative airflow rooms?

Continued on page 84

FIGURE 3-10. Sample ICRA Matrix of Precautions for Construction and Renovation, continued

Step 11. Do the plans allow for the required number and type of hand-washing sinks?

Step 12. Does the IC staff agree with the minimum number of sinks for this project? (Verify against *AIA Guidelines* for types and area.)

Step 13. Does the IC staff agree with the plans relative to clean and soiled utility rooms?

Step 14. Plan to discuss the following containment issues with the project team: traffic flow, housekeeping, debris removal (how and when).

Appendix: Identify and communicate the responsibility for project monitoring that includes IC concerns and risks. The ICRA may be modified throughout the project. Revisions must be communicated to the project manager.

Infection Control Construction Permit					
			Permit No:		
Location of Construction:			Project Start Date:		
Project Coordinator:			Estimated Duration:		
Contractor Performing Work:			Permit Expiration Date:		
Supervisor:			Telephone:		
YES	NO	CONSTRUCTION ACTIVITY	YES	NO	INFECTION CONTROL RISK GROUP
		TYPE A: Inspection, noninvasive activity			GROUP 1: Low Risk
		TYPE B: Small scale, short duration, moderate to high levels			GROUP 2: Medium Risk
		TYPE C: Activity generates moderate to high levels of dust, requires > 1 work shift for completion			GROUP 3: Medium/High Risk
		TYPE D: Major duration and construction activities requiring consecutive work shifts			GROUP 4: Highest Risk
CLASS I		1. Execute work by methods to minimize raising dust from construction operations. 2. Immediately replace any ceiling tile displaced for visual inspection. 3. Minor demolition for remodeling.			
CLASS II		1. Provide active means to prevent airborne dust from dispersing into atmosphere. 2. Water mist work surfaces to control dust while cutting. 3. Seal unused doors with duct tape. 4. Block off and seal air vents. 5. Wipe surfaces with disinfectant. 6. Contain construction waste before transport in tightly covered containers. 7. Wet mop or vacuum with HEPA–filtered vacuum before leaving work area. 8. Place dust mat at entrance and exit of work area. 9. Remove or isolate HVAC system in areas where work is being performed.			
CLASS III		1. Obtain infection control permit before construction begins. 2. Isolate HVAC system in area where work is being done to prevent contamination of the duct system. 3. Complete all critical barriers or implement control cube method before construction begins. 4. Maintain negative air pressure within work site utilizing HEPA–equipped air filtration units. 5. Do not remove barriers from work area until complete project is thoroughly cleaned by env. services dept. 6. Vacuum work with HEPA–filtered vacuums. 7. Wet mop with disinfectant. 8. Remove barrier materials carefully to minimize spreading of dirt and debris associated with construction. 9. Contain construction waste before transport in tightly covered containers. 10. Cover transport receptacles or carts. Tape covering. 11. Remove or isolate HVAC system in areas where work is being performed.			
Date					
Initial					

Continued on page 85

FIGURE 3-10. Sample ICRA Matrix of Precautions for Construction and Renovation, continued

CLASS IV	1. Obtain infection control permit before construction begins. 2. Isolate HVAC system in area where work is being done to prevent contamination of duct system. 3. Complete all critical barriers or implement control cube method before construction begins. 4. Maintain negative air pressure within work site utilizing HEPA–equipped air filtration units. 5. Seal holes, pipes, conduits, and punctures appropriately. 6. Construct anteroom and require all personnel to pass through this room so they can be vacuumed using a HEPA vacuum cleaner before leaving work site, or they can wear cloth or paper coveralls that are removed each time they leave the work site. 7. All personnel entering work site are required to wear shoe covers. 8. Do not remove barriers from work area until completed project is thoroughly cleaned by the environmental services dept. 9. Vacuum work area with HEPA–filtered vacuums. 10. Wet mop with disinfectant. 11. Remove barrier materials carefully to minimize spreading of dirt and debris associated with construction. 12. Contain construction waste before transport in tightly covered containers. 13. Cover transport receptacles or carts. Tape covering. 14. Remove or isolate HVAC system in areas where work is being done.
Date	
Initial	

Additional Requirements: Date ____________ Initials ____________ Date ____________ Initials ____________ Exceptions/Additions to this permit are noted by attached memoranda

Permit Requested By: ____________________ Permit Authorized By: ____________________

Date: ____________________ Date: ____________________

This form is only one way of conducting the infection control assessment portion of a proactive risk assessment. Organizations that choose to use this form should be aware that it does NOT include assessments of utilities, noise, vibration, air flow, and emergency procedures—items that the Joint Commission does require as part of the proactive risk assessment.

Source: Patient Safety Institute, Premier, Inc. Used with permission. Steps 1-3 adapted with permission, V. Kennedy, B. Barnard, St. Luke Episcopal Hospital, Houston, TX; C. Fine, CA. Steps 4-14 adapted with permission, Fairview University Medical Center, Minneapolis, MN. Forms modified and provided courtesy of J. Bartley, ECSI Inc., Beverly Hills, MI.

Standard EC.5.50

(AHC, BHC, CAH, HAP, LTC, OME)

The organization develops and implements activities to protect occupants during periods when a building does not meet the applicable provisions of the Life Safety Code®.

Elements of Performance

1. (AHC, BHC, CAH, HAP, LTC, OME) Each organization develops a policy for using interim life safety measures (ILSM).

2. (AHC, BHC, CAH, HAP, LTC, OME) The policy includes written criteria for evaluating various deficiencies and construction hazards to determine when and to what extent one or more of the following ILSM apply:

- *Ensuring free and unobstructed exits. Staff receive additional information/communication when alternative exits are designated. Buildings or areas under construction must maintain escape routes for construction workers at all times, and the means of exiting construction areas are inspected daily.*
- *Ensuring free and unobstructed access to emergency services and for fire, police, and other emergency forces.*
- *Ensuring that fire alarm, detection, and suppression systems are in good working order. A temporary but equivalent system must be provided when any fire system is impaired. Temporary systems must be inspected and tested monthly.**
- *Ensuring that temporary construction partitions are smoke-tight and built of noncombustible or limited combustible materials that will not contribute to the development or spread of fire.*
- *Providing additional fire-fighting equipment and training staff in its use.*
- *Prohibiting smoking throughout the [organization]'s buildings and in and near construction areas.*
- *Developing and enforcing storage, housekeeping, and debris removal practices that reduce the building's flammable and combustible fire load to the lowest feasible level.*
- *Conducting a minimum of two fire drills (BHC, CAH, HAP, LTC, OME: per shift) per quarter.*
- *Increasing surveillance of buildings, grounds, and equipment, with special attention to excavations, con-*

* The *Life Safety Code®*, NFPA 101–2000 edition, requires that the municipal fire department (or applicable emergency forces group) is notified and a fire watch is provided whenever an approved fire alarm or automatic sprinkler system is out of service for more than 4 hours in a 24-hour period in an occupied building.

struction areas, construction storage, and field offices.

• *Training staff to compensate for impaired structural or compartmentalization* features of fire safety.*

• *Conducting organizationwide safety education programs to promote awareness of fire-safety building deficiencies, construction hazards, and ILSM.*

3. (AHC, BHC, CAH, HAP, LTC, OME) Each [organization] implements ILSM as defined in its policy.

Interim Life Safety Measures

When renovation or construction activities are taking place, the safety of patients, staff, and other occupants of a facility is often compromised. Construction and renovation can involve flammable materials and "hot work" permits such as welding and soldering. In addition, fire detection, suppression, and alarm devices may be out of service, and normal exits and escape paths may be blocked. These conditions present threats to patient safety that must be addressed. Standard EC.5.50 requires organizations to develop and implement activities to protect occupants during periods when a building does not meet the applicable provisions of the *LSC*.

Before 1997, the Joint Commission required that facilities implement all 11 ILSM every time a deficiency occurred. To give health care facilities more control and flexibility, the standard has since been modified. The Joint Commission still requires that ILSM actions be taken to correct deficiencies, but facilities can now choose which of the 11 actions to implement based on the situation. The standard now mandates that each facility "develops a policy for using interim life safety measures. The policy includes written criteria for evaluating various deficiencies and construction hazards to determine when and to what extent one or more of the [ILSM] measures apply."

Appropriate ILSM should be implemented anytime a lapse in *LSC* compliance is evident, and, as previously mentioned, construction and renovation projects are ripe for such compliance violations. Common *LSC* deficiencies during construction involve the safety and accessibility of patient rooms, fire exits, EDs, and alarm and sprinkler systems.

To comply with standard EC.5.50, organizations should have a specific policy in place that determines how the organization will assess *LSC* compliance and respond to deficiencies during construction. To conduct the life safety assessment, organizations can complete the Joint Commission's Statement of Conditions™ (SOC) document. The SOC is a proactive tool that assists in providing a critical self-assessment of a facility's current level of compliance with the *LSC* and a description of how to resolve *LSC* deficiencies.

When conducting the *LSC* assessment, organizations should have a multidisciplinary team review the construction and phasing drawings of the facility and look for areas of noncompliance. This group should also determine which measures are appropriate to address identified lapses in compliance. Members of the multidisciplinary team may include the following:

- Safety officer
- Construction manager
- Facility manager
- Risk manager
- Security manager
- Administration representative
- Representative of affected staff, such as a nurse manager from the ICU if the construction project affects the ICU
- Architect
- Engineers
- Contractor and appropriate subcontractors (these would be the mechanical, electrical, and controls subcontractors)

Some organizations choose to conduct their ILSM assessment and their proactive risk assessment at the same time, using the same team. Although this is not required by the Joint Commission, it may be a helpful way to ensure that both assessments are coordinated and no critical areas are overlooked. Case Study 3-6 beginning on page 87 discusses how two organizations conducted their proactive risk assessments and ILSM assessments before a construction project.

The Joint Commission is not the only entity that requires organizations to determine ILSM for building projects. Most states require organizations to submit applicable ILSM when they submit their project drawings.

By its very nature, an ILSM is intended to be temporary. It should be in place only while the compliance lapse exists. After an organization comes back into compliance with the *LSC*, the ILSM can be eliminated. Therefore, if an organization is taking a phased approach to a construction process, it needs to implement the ILSM during the phase in which the *LSC* lapse is present. Each time there is an *LSC* lapse, an ILSM must be implemented.

* **Compartmentalization** The concept of using various building components (fire walls and doors, smoke barriers, fire-rated floor slabs, and so forth) to prevent the spread of fire and the production's combustion, and to provide a safe means of egress to an approved exit. The presence of these features varies depending upon the building occupancy classification.

Case Study 3-6. Standardizing the Assessment of Life Safety and Infection Control Risks

Two Organizations Take a Comprehensive Approach to Addressing Safety Risks in Construction

Elmhurst Memorial Healthcare

Like most hospitals around the country, Elmhurst Memorial Healthcare, located in Elmhurst, Illinois, has multiple construction, renovation, and redecorating projects going at any one time. With 427 licensed beds and a staff of 3,200 employees and 600 physicians, the organization has many lives to consider when assessing safety risks involved with construction. To ensure the safety of all its construction projects, Elmhurst Memorial created a standardized process for assessing life safety and IC issues. This process was created by Dave Samples, facilities engineer, and Cari Cooper, R.N., C.I.C., for Elmhurst Memorial Healthcare.

At the start of construction projects, the organization reviews its compliance with the *LSC* and determines ILSM for the construction period. It also reviews IC issues and selects control measures to address them. The organization uses ILSM and IC grid worksheets to aid in this process. The facility engineer uses one worksheet to evaluate the ILSM. (*See* Figure 3-11 on page 88.) He circles all issues on the grid that apply to the particular construction project. He then adds up the associated points to get a total score for the project. Depending on the number of points, different ILSM are required to be implemented. The ILSM are decided on and posted on bright red posters that are hung at all construction entrances. (*See* Figure 4-2 in Chapter Four.)

For IC, the facility engineer completes the IC measures evaluation worksheet to assess IC issues. (*See* Figure 3-12 on page 89.) Again, the facility engineer circles the applicable information, adds up the points, and determines the necessary control measures based on the total number of points. As with the ILSM, the organization uses a standardized list of control measures based on the different point ranges. (*See* Figure 3-13 on page 90.) In addition to the facility engineer, the Infection Control Practitioner must sign off on the IC worksheet before construction begins. After the worksheet is filled out, the ICRA measures that are implemented are posted on bright pink posters and hung at each construction areas entrance.

"We created the ILSM grid about 10 years ago," says Dave Samples, facilities engineer for Elmhurst Memorial Healthcare. "We used the NFPA as a resource and assigned points based on their standards. The grid worked so well for ILSM, we decided to create one for infection control risk assessments too. They allow for staff to also be aware and monitor compliance too. In addition, daily inspections by Facilities Management and Infection Control Practitioners are conducted to monitor compliance."

To review and coordinate all the construction projects, Elmhurst has weekly construction meetings. These meetings include representatives from the following areas:

- Facilities
- Security
- Environmental Services
- Infection Control
- Architects
- Engineers
- Contractors
- Manager for the area under construction
- Clinical staff
- Physicians

During these meetings, the group evaluates and discusses any ILSM and IC measures planned or underway.

Other issues, such as noise and vibration, are dealt with on a case-by-case basis in regular construction meetings between the architect, engineering staff, IS group, and the clinical groups. "Each project is so different that we haven't yet come up with a universal grid to address these issues," notes Samples.

St. Alphonsus Regional Medical Center

Like Elmhurst Memorial Healthcare, St. Alphonsus Regional Medical Center, a 381-bed medical/surgical acute care facility located in Boise, Idaho, created a standardized process for assessing life safety issues. Prior to construction, the project manager completes a safety assessment form (*see* Figure 3-14 on page 91) and the plant

Continued on page 88

Continued from page 87

FIGURE 3-11. INTERIM LIFE SAFETY MEASURES EVALUATION WORKSHEET

Criteria:					
Job Length	> 3 Months: (40)	1–3 Months (25)	< 1 Month (15)	< 2 Weeks (10)	< 1 Week (0)
Impact on Patient Care	Inpatient Care Area (40)	Ambulatory Care Area (30)	Visitors, & Staff (25)	Staff Only (10)	Unoccupied (0)
Hazards of Construction Materials	Flammable Materials (50)		Combustible Materials (40)		Low-Hazard Materials (0)
Hazards Of Construction Methods	Open Flames, Flame Welding (50)		Heat Producing Electric Welding (40)		Low-Hazard Methods Only (0)
Fire and Smoke Separations	Separation Missing (40)	Big Holes or Gaps (30)	Minor Holes, Penetrations (20)	1–2 Minor Penetrations (10)	Separation Intact –1 Hour (0)
Impact On Exiting	Exits Blocked, > 2 Exits (50)	Exit Obstruction, 2 Exits (35)	Exit Stair Penetrations (25)		No Obstruction (0)
Impact On Exit Access	< 2 Exits, Inadequate Exits (50)	Redirect or Reroute Exiting (35)		Excess Travel Distance (10)	No Exit Impact (0)
Impact On Fire Alarm & Sprinkler Systems	Multiple Zones or System Disabled (40)	Single Zone Disabled, or Affected (25)		Work on Fire Alarm System Disables (10)	System Fully Operational (0)
Temporary Construction Partitions	Partitions Not Smoke Tight, Fire Rated 1 Hour (50)	Multiple Partitions (40)	Single Partition (30)	Minor Penetrations (25)	No Openings/ Partition Smoke and Fire Rated for 1 Hour (0)
Storage Areas	Multiple Storage in Zone (40)	One Storage in Zone (25)	Storage in Adjacent Areas (25)		No Storage on Floor (0)
Access to Building & Exterior	Blocked or Obstructed exits (50)	Single Exit Discharge Blocked (50)	Building Exterior. Obstructed > 75′ (35)		No Obstruction Along Building (0)

TOTAL POINTS = PERSON - DATE / /

FINAL SCORING IMPACT A total score of more than

50–95 generally represents an indication of the need to do Interim Life Safety Measures (ILSM) with daily fire watches.

100–245 is an indication of ILSM with hourly fire watches.

250–500 is an indication of ILSM with a 24 hour & 7 days a week permanent fire watch.

Elmhurst uses this worksheet to evaluate the need for ILSM.

Source: Elmhurst Memorial Healthcare, Elmhurst, IL.

Continued on page 89

Continued from page 88

FIGURE 3-12. Infection Control Measures Evaluation Worksheet

Criteria:					
Job Length	>3 Months: (30)	1–3 Months (25)	< 1 Month (15)	1 Week (5)	< 1 Week (0)
Impact on Patient Care	High-Risk Patient Care Area (50)	General Patient Care Area (40)	Visitors, & Staff Area (20)	Staff Only (10)	Unoccupied Area (0)
Hazards of Construction Work	Water Damage Demolition (50)	Major Demolition (40)	General Construction (20)	Decorating, Minor Work (10)	General Maintenance (0)
Hazards Of Construction Methods	Wallboard & Plaster Demolition (50)	Carpet & Ceiling Demolition (40)	Millwork & Other Demolition (20)	Mounting, Drilling, etc. (10)	Low-Hazard Methods Only (0)
Construction Separations	Separation Missing (50)	Big Holes or Gaps (30)	Plastic Sheets to Ceiling (10)	Separate Room w/ Door (5)	Wall Separation & Airtight (0)
Ventilation Pressure	Positive Pressure (50)	Neutral Pressure & Outside Exhaust (30)	Neutral Pressure & HEPA (20)	Negative & Outside Exhaust (10)	HEPA & Negative Pressure (0)
Other Controls	None (50)	Sticky Entrance Mats (30)	Mats, HEPA Vacuum, Daily Mopping (20)	Mats, Vacuum, Mop, No Trash (10)	Mats, HEPA Vacuum, Mopping, No Trash, & All Vents Sealed (0)

Evaluation Performed by - **Date -** / /

Infection Control Approval - **Date -** / /

Project Name -

FINAL SCORE =______________ (see next page for temporary measures to be implemented)

Elmhurst Memorial Healthcare uses this worksheet to evaluate the need for infection control measures.

Source: Elmhurst Memorial Healthcare, Elmhurst, IL.

Continued on page 90

Continued from page 89

FIGURE 3-13 Temporary IC Control Measures for Implementation

TEMPORARY CONTROL MEASURES FOR IMPLEMENTATION

Based on the final score obtained from the evaluation the following control measures should be taken, as needed. Infection control measures implemented as a result of the ICRA will then be indicated on the posting notice (see attachment # 1), and will be posted on bright pink paper next to the red ILSM posting notices at all entrances to any worksites.

SCORE OF 250 – 350 "HIGH RISK"

(check if applicable)

_____- HEPA Filter Unit
_____- Negative Pressure (with supplies blocked and returns filtered with HEPA media)
_____- Negative Pressure (with outside exhaust)
_____- Temporary Airtight Walls (slab to slab 1 hour rating)
_____- Sticky Floor Mats at Entrances
_____- Anteroom Required
_____- Daily HEPA Vacuuming of Site
_____- Daily Mopping of Site by Environmental Services
_____- All Supply and Return Vents Sealed Off (neutral pressure)
_____- Daily Removal of All Trash (in covered containers)
_____- Monitoring of Patients in Project Area for Infection
_____- Close All Doors to Patient Care Areas in the Vicinity of the Work Area
_____- Coveralls Used in All Work Areas & Removed upon Leaving the Work Site

SCORE OF 150 – 250 "MEDIUM RISK"

_____- Temporary Airtight Walls or Fire-Rated Plastic Sheeting (only to ceiling if ceiling is intact)
_____- Supply and Return Vents Sealed Off (neutral pressure)
_____- Sticky Floor Mats at Entrances
_____- Daily HEPA Vacuuming of Site
_____- Daily Floor Mopping of Site by Environmental Services
_____- Daily Trash Removal
_____- Close All Doors in the Vicinity of the Work Site

SCORE OF 50 – 150 "LOW RISK"

_____- Temporary Fire-Rated Plastic Sheeting
_____- Daily Trash Removal
_____- Daily HEPA Vacuuming of Site
_____- Close All Doors to the Work Site

PROJECT CLEANUP AND DISPOSAL

- Barriers cannot be removed from the work area until Facilities Management inspects the completed project and the area is thoroughly cleaned. After removal and a final contractor cleanup, a final disinfecting will be performed by Environmental Services who will be notified of construction completion time one week ahead.
- Work area must be vacuumed with HEPA–filtered vacuums.
- Wet mop area with disinfectant.
- Remove barrier materials carefully to minimize spreading dust and debris.
- Barriers used should be treated as debris and disposed of accordingly.
- Construction waste must be either bagged or transported in covered carts.
- Remove blockage of air vents.

Source: Elmhurst Memorial Healthcare, Elmhurst, IL.

Continued on page 91

Continued from page 90

FIGURE 3-14 Safety Assessment

Saint Alphonsus Regional Medical Center
Renovation/Construction/Life Safety/Safety Assessment

Project (Designation from Plans) ______________________________

Item ____________________ Start Date _______ End Date _______

1. Will normal egress routes or exits be obstructed by renovation? ❑ Yes ❑ No
If yes, list location(s).

2. Will fire alarm, detection, or suppression systems be impaired? ❑ Yes ❑ No
List systems and length of downtime.

3. Will existing smoke barriers or fire walls be compromised? ❑ Yes ❑ No
If yes, list location(s).

4. Will hazardous or flammable materials be brought on site? ❑ Yes ❑ No
If yes, list below and attach MSDS for all materials.

5. Will renovation affect more than one department? ❑ Yes ❑ No
If yes, list departments.

6. Please indicate type of construction. ❑ Yes ❑ No

TYPE A: Inspection, noninvasive activity
TYPE B: Small scale, short duration, moderate to high levels
TYPE C: Generates moderate to high levels of dust, requires greater than 1 work shift for completion
TYPE D: Major duration and construction activities requiring consecutive work shifts

7. Will utility or security systems be impaired? ❑ Yes ❑ No
If yes, list systems and estimated downtime.

Project Coordinator____________________ Date ___________

Source: St. Alphonsus Regional Medical Center, Boise, ID.

Continued on page 92

Continued from page 91

FIGURE 3-15 ILSM Compliance Plan

Saint Alphonsus Regional Medical Center
Interim Life Safety Management (ILSM) Compliance Plan

1. Staff Training	Contractor	Renovation Department	Facility-wide	N/A
a. Alternative evacuation routes.				
b. Alternative exits and passageways.				
c. Fire system deficiencies.				
d. Alternative fire protection equipment.				
e. Use of fire protection equipment.				
f. Location of temporary barriers.				
g. Storage of hazardous or flammable materials.				
h. Additional fire drills (___ per month).				
i. Smoking policy.				
j. Other.				

2. Hazard Surveillance	Daily	Alternate Days	Weekly	Bi-Weekly
a. Means of egress in construction.				
b. Storage of hazardous or flammable materials.				
c. Departments adjacent to renovation.				
d. Safety department inspections.				
e. Signage identifying construction.				

3. Modifications to Work Area	YES	NO	Comments
a. Additional signage required? ❑ Construction warning ❑ Exit maps ❑ Fire protection equipment ❑ Special hazards			
b. Additional fire protection required?			
c. Fire watch need to be established?			
d. Smoke proof partition needed?			
e. Flammable liquid storage needed?			
f. Security needed in the area?			

Safety Officer ______________________________

Source: St. Alphonsus Regional Medical Center, Boise, ID.

Continued on page 93

Continued from page 92

operations manager, safety manager, and the infection control practitioner review it. The form addresses ILSM issues, including the following:

- Egress routes and exits
- Fire alarm, detection, and suppression systems
- Smoke barriers
- Hazardous flammable materials
- Security

To assess IC issues, St. Alphonsus uses the previously mentioned ICRA form, developed by the Patient Safety Institute (*see* page 81–85). The organization's IC professional is assigned responsibility for completing the form and ensuring the implementation of control measures. To complete the form, the IC professional examines a project description and participates in a meeting with the project manager about the nature, scope, and risks associated with the project.

Issues about noise, vibration, and the like are discussed at the outset with the project manager. "Some issues may need to go to security for approval," says William Morgan, manager of plant operations and facility engineering for St. Alphonsus. "We also discuss what systems may need to have emergency response plans and we assign responsibility."

Other safety issues that St. Alphonsus considers before construction begins include the following:

- Patient, staff, visitor, and construction parking
- Eating on the construction site
- Contractor access to the facility
- Patient privacy

"It's important to discuss these issues with the contractor before the start of construction. This helps minimize confusion and ensures a safe building process," says Morgan.

After construction begins, both these organizations ensure that control measures are properly implemented and actively monitor the construction site for further safety risks. (*See* the second part of this case study in Chapter Four, beginning on page 110.)

CASE AT A GLANCE

■ Main challenge
To create a streamlined, integrated assessment process for IC and other safety risks and ILSM.

■ Issues
Significant risks to patients exist during the construction process. Organizations must assess and address these risks.

■ Solutions
Elmhurst Memorial Healthcare created worksheets to help with the assessment process and developed standardized responses based on a quantified level of risk. St. Alphonsus also uses an assessment form to determine ILSM and IC risks and works with the general contractor to deal with noise, vibration, and other issues.

■ Outcomes
Both organizations successfully prepare for construction projects and address any risks involved.

Survey Considerations

If an organization is in the midst of a construction or renovation project at the time of its triennial survey, the Joint Commission does not want the organization to cease work because of the survey. In fact, the Joint Commission expects that any construction or renovation work will continue throughout the survey process.

Some areas related to construction and renovation that surveyors may look at during survey include the following:

- General safety issues
- ILSM—This will include the assessment of *LSC* compliance and implementation of ILSM
- Proactive risk assessment—This will include how the assessment is done, the scope of the assessment (including ICRAs), and the continuity with the ILSM assessment
- Cleanliness of the construction site
- Appropriate behavior of construction workers
- Perspective of staff. Surveyors may ask staff members in nearby compartments how long the construction will last and how they are affected by construction efforts.

The planning, design, and construction process is a journey with many twists and turns. At some point along the way, an organization may have questions or concerns about the process and the Joint Commission's requirements regarding the process. As with other compliance issues, the Joint Commission is happy to answer any questions about planning, design, and construction. Organizations should contact the Standards Interpretation Group with any questions or concerns.

SIDEBAR 3-10.
Extension Surveys

The Joint Commission may need to conduct an extension survey of an organization, if the organization has done the following:

- Instituted a new service or program for which the Joint Commission has standards
- Changed ownership with a significant number of changes in the management and clinical staff or operating policies and procedures
- Offered at least 25% of its services at a new location or in a significantly altered physical plant
- Expanded its capacity to provide services by 25% or more as measured by patient volume, pieces of equipment, or other relevant measures
- Provided a more intensive level of service

or

- Merged with, consolidated with, or acquired an unaccredited site, service, or program for which there are applicable Joint Commission standards and EPs

An extension survey is conducted at an accredited organization or at a site that is owned and operated by the organization, if the accredited organization's current accreditation is not due to expire for at least nine months and when at least one of the conditions above is met. The results of an extension survey may affect the organization's accreditation decision.

REFERENCES

1. Leonard M., Frankel A., Simmonds T.: *Achieving Safe and Reliable Healthcare,* Chicago: Heath Administration Press, 2004.

2. Carlson School of Management: *Designing a Safe Hospital* Publication 1 Series. Minneapolis: University of Minnesota, 2002.

3. Reiling J., et al.: FMEA: The cure for medical errors. *Quality Progress* 36:67–71, Aug. 2003.

4. Telephone interview with Karen Lambert, CEO, and Roseanne Niese, director of emergency, intensive care, and nursing resource services, of Advocate Good Shepherd Hospital, Barrington, IL. May 2005.

5. Joint Commission Resources: Designing for improved patient flow: Structuring space helps keep patients moving. *Environment of Care News* 7:8–10, May 2004.

6. Sandrick K.: Designing a defense: Using architectural elements to help reduce contact infection risks. *Healthcare Facilities Management,* May 2002.

7. Joint Commission Resources: Building in infection control from the ground up: Northwestern Memorial Hospital fights infection by design. *Environment of Care News* 7:8–10, Oct. 2004.

8. Bartley, J.M.: APIC state-of-the-art report: The role of infection control during construction in health care facilities. *Am J Infect Control* 28:156–169, Apr. 2000.

9. Telephone interview with William Morgan, manager of plant operations and facility engineering for St. Alphonsus Regional Medical Center, Boise, ID, Jun. 2005.

10. American Institute of Architects (AIA): *Guidelines for Design and Construction of Hospital and Health Care Facilities.* Washington, DC, AIA, 2001.

11. Old L.: Construction risk management. Paper presented at the ASHE International Conference and Exhibition on Health Facility Planning Design and Construction, Chicago, Mar. 7, 2005.

12. Telephone interview with Dave Samples, facilities engineer for Elmhurst Memorial Healthcare, Elmhurst, IL, Jun. 2005.

CHAPTER FOUR:

Building Design and Construction

ALTHOUGH A LARGE PORTION of the planning, design, and construction journey involves planning, at one point the organization must commit to a design, put it on paper, and construct the project. That is not to say there can't be changes or alterations to the project; however, the later along the way these changes are made, the more they are likely to cost.

The design phase is somewhat fluid and still requires the participation and input of organization leadership and staff. The construction process is less fluid than design, but organizations can still encounter issues along the way that will alter the best-laid plans. The following sections can help organizations navigate the building design and construction processes.

Schematic Design

The primary goal of schematic design is to create a clearly defined, feasible design concept, a preliminary construction schedule, and a preliminary construction budget. Schematic design is the point at which the overall scope of the project is tested and confirmed.

During schematic design, the project's overall configuration and organization of component parts (buildings, departments, floor levels, and functional areas or zones) should be established, along with building and site circulation patterns. In schematic drawings, the building is located on the site, along with key features such as parking and entry points. Overall building materials and systems, such as exterior cladding materials and structural/mechanical systems, should be selected during this phase. All these elements are brought together to establish a holistic creative vision and give the project its overall image and form.

The Process Involved

Often, the creative process is not linear, particularly with complex design problems. The architect and consultant team tests many ideas and develops alternatives. Schematic design is the time for testing alternatives, when the project team works together to identify the best overall design solutions. Team participation is critical because this is usually the first opportunity for organization leadership and key facility staff to understand the spatial implications of their planning efforts.

Not only is schematic design the time when an overall design concept is developed and evaluated, it is also the appropriate time to initiate regulatory agency involvement and review.

At the end of schematic design, documentation should communicate all design decisions to date in a format that can be visualized, understood, and evaluated. This documentation includes three-dimensional information (renderings and models), two-dimensional information (floor plans), narrative information (preliminary specifications), and tabular information (a space list, construction budget, and project schedule).

Design Drawings and Models

Drawings and models are the architect's tools for creative exploration and the exchange of design ideas with others involved in the process. These materials are frequently used to make public presentations for fundraising and promotional purposes. Drawings developed in a schematic design can also facilitate coordination with consultants and engineers, builders or contractors, and regulatory agencies. These drawings and models are produced at a scale that clearly illustrates the overall concept. Following are some typical types of schematic design drawings:

Site plans. These drawings include the entire property. They illustrate the location and layout of existing and proposed buildings, roads, parking, utilities, property lines, zoning setbacks, easements, land contours, and other features of the site design. They may include tabular information on building and parking areas and narrative descriptions of zoning constraints.

Floor plans. These illustrate the layout of each floor or level for each building. The amount of detail may vary depending on the size of the project. Each room, space, or area in the building program is placed and identified. Door and window sizes and locations are shown (unless the project is so large that the scale of the drawings does not allow for clear communication of this information). Floor plans at the schematic design stage usually include overall building dimensions.

Building exterior elevations. These illustrate the appearance, size, and shape of significant exterior building walls or vertical elements. They indicate the grade and slope of the ground at the building face; door and window sizes and locations; roof profiles;

and other significant design elements. These drawings include overall (vertical) dimensions and floor elevations.

Building sections. At this stage building sections usually illustrate typical building conditions and special volumetric conditions, such as the view through an atrium or lobby. These drawings indicate the exterior wall or "skin" profile, floor locations and heights, floor/ceiling and wall thicknesses, and other important cross-sectional information.

Preliminary specifications. Specifications at the schematic design phase are intended to provide a general description of the work, including major building components and systems (civil, structural, architectural, mechanical, electrical, and plumbing), as well as basic materials selection. Significant materials and systems are identified but not described in detail. This document is often in the form of a narrative.

Revised building program or space list. This tabular information is presented as a revision of the building program prepared during predesign or master planning. It may be formatted in a manner that allows for comparison of programmed area versus proposed schematic design area on a room-by-room, departmental, or overall building area basis.

At the conclusion of the schematic design stage, a direction should be chosen from the options proposed by the design team, which will be developed further in the next phase.

Design Development

The primary objective of design development is to develop preliminary design ideas into a more detailed, complete understanding and presentation of the design proposal. All elements established in the schematic design are studied in greater detail, and more detailed elements are studied, selected, and designed.

By the completion of design development, all significant components of the project should be identified, defined, described, sized, and located. This detailed design information must be prepared in a format that all project team members can understand and approve. This is critical to the project delivery schedule because failure to effectively communicate this information can cause frustration, delay, and added expense later. As a result of the design development process, all project team members should have a common, detailed understanding of the project scope and design intent.

Design development begins after the organization has signed off on the schematic design proposal. Some of the details design development addresses include individual spaces, rooms, component assemblies, building systems, and material selections. In an interactive planning and design process, organization leadership and staff are involved with making recommendations and providing feedback on detailed design elements. Ideally, this exchange is an extension of the programming and planning process started during master planning and predesign.

Extensive interaction occurs between architects, structural engineers, mechanical engineers, electrical engineers, and other project consultants during design development. Frequent and effective communication is essential to coordinate the detailed design of interrelated building systems, assemblies, and equipment among the firms and individuals responsible for each area.

Some important aspects of the design development process include the following:

Space planning. Space planning involves determining the way a given space will be furnished, organized, and equipped. It may be provided or directed by the architect, an independent planning consultant, health care facility staff, or any combination thereof. As mentioned in Chapter Three, organizations should consider standardizing patient rooms to enhance safety and efficiency. Space plans should reflect such standardization.

Interior design. The detailed design of building interiors also begins during design development. Interior design services involve the selection and coordination of interior finish materials, material colors, signage and graphic design, and furniture. These services may include the procurement of interior furnishings. As mentioned previously, organizations should keep in mind infection control, fire and smoke ratings, and safety when selecting finish materials. In addition, organizations should pay close attention to colors, signage, and graphic designs to ensure that he building promotes a healing environment.

Medical equipment planning. Organizations should have begun discussions about medical equipment during the master planning/predesign phase. Ideally, the planning team developed a list of potential equipment. At the design development phase, the design team needs to know types, sizes, and supporting service requirements of equipment to fully define the spaces intended to accommodate major pieces of fixed and movable equipment. Medical equipment planning is a specialty in itself. Relatively few architectural firms maintain the internal resources and ongoing expertise for substantive equipment planning and selection. Typically, an equipment planning consultant provides this service, contracting directly with the organization.

By the end of design development, the type and location of materials and systems should be easily seen in the documentation provided by the design team. This enables development of a revised, more detailed project schedule and budget.

Assigning Equipment Costs

The assignment of major equipment costs to either the construction budget or other capital expense categories is a key issue. Equipment provided and installed under the construction contract should be included in the construction budget. Major medical equipment that is purchased and installed under separate contracts should be identified as a separate line item in the project budget. In major medical equipment construction budgeting, the cost of preparing the architectural, structural, mechanical, electrical, and plumbing systems becomes part of the construction budget, but the organization retains responsibility for procurement and installation.

Regulatory Review

Although most organizations will begin to involve regulatory agencies and "authorities having jurisdiction" during the schematic design stage, design development activities should also include ongoing involvement of local zoning officials and building inspectors, as well as state regulatory agencies. It is important to keep regulatory officials abreast of design decisions early and often to avoid regulatory problems and redesign. Organizations should also involve insurance agencies at this time.

Documentation

Design development documentation builds on the information contained in schematic design documents. This documentation provides a detailed representation of the project that can be understood and approved by the organization and used to coordinate with project consultants and contractors. It establishes the design baseline that will become a guide for the preparation of construction documentation. It also provides a thorough documentation of project scope and complexity for estimating purposes.

Graphic documentation at design development should include revised versions of materials presented at the conclusion of the schematic design phase, along with a great deal of new information. It should have much greater detail and be drawn at a larger scale. Additional models or renderings should be provided to communicate key elements or spaces in the project to the organization leadership and staff as well as to the public.

Following are some common types of design development drawings:

Site plans. Site plans indicate all the information provided at the schematic design, but are revised to reflect design changes and a more detailed design solution. Site plans for phased projects identify the scope and location of each project phase. Grading and site elevations are identified in detail. Surface materials and landscape design proposals are also represented.

Building floor plans. These plans are provided for all floors or levels in the project, as in the schematic design. They are revised to illustrate the current status of design and are at a larger scale than plans presented in the schematics. Each space indicates door and window widths, door swing direction, built-in cabinets and counters, plumbing fixtures, and major equipment layouts. Wall thicknesses are accurately portrayed. Each space is labeled, or keyed to a legend, to identify room names and numbers.

Exterior building elevations. Elevations illustrate all exterior building faces and include an update of information presented at schematic design and show greater detail. Exterior materials and the configuration of exterior building elements are also illustrated in detail. At times, this detailed information is portrayed in enlarged elevation drawings that represent typical portions of the facade showing items such as brick patterns, window or door trim configurations, and so on.

Building sections. Building sections are enlargements and revisions of building sections developed during the schematic design stage. They illustrate design changes and a greater level of development. These drawings identify and distinguish structural elements, mechanical spaces, interior and exterior wall/floor profiles, and interior space configurations.

Reflected ceiling plans. These plans illustrate the ceiling surface of interior spaces and are drawn at the same scale as corresponding floor plans. Their purpose is to indicate the layout, size, and profile of all ceiling systems and ceiling-mounted fixtures. These plans include light fixture types and patterns, other ceiling-mounted equipment, lay-in ceiling grid patterns, changes in ceiling height, and so forth.

Enlarged floor plans. These floor plans are keyed to building floor plans and are developed for the detailed study and presentation of important, complex spaces, such as patient rooms, diagnostic and treatment areas, operating rooms, and others. The plans are used to coordinate and illustrate space planning, equipment planning, and furniture layouts in response to functional criteria and other human needs for the space. Room standardization should be apparent in these enlarged floor plans.

Interior elevations. Interior elevations are prepared for spaces represented in enlarged floor plans and major public areas of the building interior. They illustrate detailed information, such as cabinets and other millwork, interior windows and other openings, wall surface details, equipment mounting locations, plumbing fixture arrangements, medical gas outlet locations, and so on.

Typical wall sections. Wall sections are created to illustrate highly repetitive or common wall types. They can illustrate interior and exterior wall assemblies for cost-estimating purposes.

Equipment plans. These are plan drawings limited to illustrating the layout and size of major medical, food service, reprocessing, or other kinds of equipment. They are prepared by the consultants contracted for equipment planning and in some cases by the equipment vendor. Plans for specific equipment types may be prepared by different consultants.

Life safety drawings. These will visually represent how the organization complies with the *Life Safety Code®** (*LSC*). Contents of such drawings will include fire walls, smoke barriers, corridors, and exits, as applicable.

Room Data Sheets

Many health facility rooms and spaces have extensive requirements for specific equipment, furnishings, heating and air-conditioning, electrical, plumbing, medical gas, and communication systems. These requirements need to be determined, recorded, and communicated to appropriate members of the project design and construction teams in a timely and detailed manner. The room data sheet (*see* Figure 4-1 on page 102) is the standard format for recording the requirements of clinical and patient care areas. The room data sheet can be prepared in several ways, depending on who is responsible for documentation. Typically, room data identifies the type, scope, and location of all necessary room elements and systems on a single sheet for each room. The sheet may also identify who will be responsible for purchase and installation (or this may be done as a separate document for the overall project). Determining and documenting room data may be a joint effort of health care facility staff, an equipment consultant, and the architect, or it may be prepared entirely by health care facility staff. The room data sheet should reflect any standardization desired between rooms.

Room Mock-ups

Full-size mock-ups of key patient care or treatment spaces often are built, usually in unoccupied on-site space, unleased commercial space, or nearby warehouses. Mock-ups are normally made of metal or wood stud framing with gypsum board or plywood wall surfaces. Mock-ups simulate the functional and spatial characteristics of the proposed room, complete with representations of cabinet work, furniture, equipment, plumbing and lighting fixtures, electrical and medical gas outlets, communications outlets, and so forth. They can be indispensable tools for communicating the reality of space to the staff who will work there. Staff can, in effect, "test drive" the space to ensure that it accommodates its intended functions. This, in turn, allows staff members to make informed recommendations for necessary design changes or improvements. Many organizations use these mock-ups to ensure a safety-focused design that addresses infection control, as well as ergonomic and security considerations. All staff members who will use the room should be encouraged to provide feedback on the room layout and design.

Mock-up rooms can also be used for simulation of current or redesigned processes. The processes can be routine, such as medication delivery in a patient room, or complex, such as those involved in an emergency code. Mock-up rooms can also be used for planning for education and orientation. Using the mock-up rooms for training until the completion of the remodeled or new space can be useful in minimizing transition errors.[1]

Revising the Budget and Schedule

The design development phase describes project construction content to a point that allows for detailed budgeting. Qualified builders or cost estimators can estimate the size and quantity of most significant building materials fairly accurately from a well-prepared set of design development drawings. They can quantify major equipment, special construction sys-

* Life Safety Code® is a registered trademark of the National Fire Protection Association, Quincy, MA.

FIGURE 4-1. Sample Room Data Sheet

Sample Room Data Sheet

Project: ____________ **Project Number:** ____________

Room Data Sheet

Date: ________

Department ____________
Room Name ____________
Net Area ____________ SF

Room Finishes
Floor ____________
Base ____________
Walls ____________
Ceiling ____________

Special Construction
Radiation Shielding ____________
Electrical Shielding ____________
Acoustical ____________
Other ____________

HVAC
Air Conditioning ____________
Air Pressure ____________
Positive ____________
Negative ____________
Outside Exhaust ____________

Plumbing Fixtures
Lavatory ____________
Water Closet ____________
Urinal ____________
Sink ____________
Sink in Counter ____________
Clinic Service Sink ____________
Tub ____________
Shower ____________
Mop Receptor ____________
Drinking Fountain ____________
Other ____________

Special Piped Utilities
Compressed Air ____________
Gas ____________
Cold Water ____________
Other ____________

Location ____________
Room Number ____________
Minimum Dimensions ____________

Medical Gas Outlets
Air ____________
Oxygen ____________
Vacuum ____________
Nitrous Oxide ____________

Lighting
General ____________
Bed Light ____________
Night Light ____________
Dimmers ____________

Power
Task Light ____________
Convenience Outlet ____________
Special Equipment Outlet ____________
X-Ray Outlet ____________
Clock Outlet ____________
TV Outlet ____________
Timer ____________
Other ____________

Communications
Telephone Outlet ____________
Nurse Call ____________
Computer Terminal ____________
Intercom ____________
Other ____________

Casework LF
Base Cabinets ____________
Wall Cabinets ____________
Countertop ____________
Open Storage Shelving ____________
Special ____________

Equipment and Additional Information ____________

This figure illustrates a room data sheet.

tems, and mechanical, electrical, and plumbing materials and systems. Construction budgets should still include contingencies; however, contingencies can be reduced to reflect more detailed understanding of the project. The allowance for inflation also should be updated and refined.

The project schedule also requires updating at the end of design development to reflect revisions to the project scope, changes in construction start dates, and a better understanding of the complexity and duration of the construction effort.

The Proactive Risk and ILSM Assessments

After the design development phase is complete, a multidisciplinary team should conduct the proactive risk assessment and the interim life safety measures (ILSM) assessment to determine any life safety, infection control, utilities, air quality, emergency management, noise, and vibration issues. Plans to address these issues should be determined at this time so control measures can be communicated to the contractor during the next phase.

Construction Documents

Also called *contract documents,* these drawings, specifications, and general contract conditions serve as the basis for a legally binding agreement between the organization and the contractor for the construction of a specific building, within a specific cost and time frame. The primary goal of this phase is to define and describe the materials, systems, assemblies, and configuration of all components and conditions of the project so that the total body of construction documents forms a well-defined scope of work. This information allows the contractor to quantify materials and labor and determine the means of constructing the project, its cost, and the amount of time needed to build it.

Typically, the preparation of construction documents begins after the owner has approved design development documentation. Contract documents are organized into three major categories: drawings, specifications, and conditions of the contract.

Drawings

Construction drawings focus on describing the scope and complexity of the design. They are visual images that identify and illustrate the location, configuration, assembly, and size of all project components. These drawings depict an integrated construction intent and do not distinguish between various suppliers, trades, or subcontractors. They include the information developed in design development but in much greater detail, as well as additional detailed information. Additional documentation is prepared in the form of detailed plan and cross-section drawings, additional enlarged plan and elevation drawings, schedules of materials, and so on. Most construction drawings are computer generated, printed, and bound in a large-sheet format. Drawings are organized into basic sections by content and intent. This enables the contractor and tradespeople to assess and understand the various elements of the work to be done. Some common components of construction drawings include the following:

Title sheet. This sheet includes an index, general project information, locator map, and building and zoning classification data; it may also include a rendering of the project.

Phasing and demolition plans. These plans include drawings that illustrate the scope of distinct construction phases in multiphased projects and areas to be demolished, renovated, and newly constructed.

Life safety plans. Life safety plans include building floor plans showing fire exit and exit access corridor locations, length of travel to exits, and location and size of fire zones or smoke compartments.

Civil/landscaping plans. These plans are site plans and drawings illustrating site utilities, excavation, grading, landscaping, and other nonarchitectural site improvements.

Architectural drawings. Architectural drawings include an architectural site plan, building floor plans, exterior building elevations, building sections, reflected ceiling plans, enlarged plans, wall sections, plan and section details, various material schedules, and interior wall elevations.

Equipment drawings. These drawings include plans and details to illustrate the scope, location, and installation details for fixed equipment to be installed or furnished under the construction contract.

Structural drawings. Structural drawings include floor plans, sections, material schedules, and details illustrating structural elements of foundation, floor, roof, wall systems, and miscellaneous structural elements.

Plumbing plans. These plans include floor/ceiling plan drawings, distribution and layout diagrams, details and plumbing fixture schedules (riser diagrams) for all plumbing systems, including water supply, waste, medical gases, and vacuum.

HVAC drawings. Heating, ventilating, and air-conditioning (HVAC) drawings include floor/ceiling plan drawings, details, and schedules illustrating the location, layout, and size of mechanical distribution equipment, systems, and devices, including air distribution ductwork, heated/chilled water pipe, and steam lines.

Electrical plans. These plans include floor/ceiling plan drawings, wiring diagrams, details, and schedules illustrating the location, layout, size, and type of electrical service distribution equipment, systems, light fixtures, outlets, switches, and other devices, including lighting, primary power, emergency power, and low-voltage systems.

Communication drawings. Communication drawings include floor/ceiling plan drawings, wiring diagrams, details, and schedules illustrating the location, layout, size, and type of electronic communication equipment, systems, outlets, and other devices; these can include telephone, nurse call, monitoring, surveillance, computer networks, cable TV, and so on.

Fire protection drawings. These drawings include floor/ceiling plan drawings, distribution and layout diagrams, details and schedules for all sprinkler and fire suppression equipment and systems, including piping, sprinkler head locations, fire department standpipe connections, exit signs, and fire hose locations.

Specifications

Specifications, found in the project specifications manual, are the detailed written data about a structure's materials, products, and systems. They range from the details of the HVAC system to the kind of window glass and door knobs used in a building. A building's specifications are contained in its project specifications manual, developed by architects, specifiers, and engineers. Contractors use the project specifications manual to bid on the project, and the winning bidder uses this manual to construct the building.[2] Architects and engineers may wish to structure their material specifications based on the 50 specification divisions developed by the Construction Specifications Institute (CSI) (*see* Sidebar 4-1).

Including ILSM and Preconstruction Risk Assessment Documents

Many organizations include the preconstruction risk assessment and ILSM assessment with the contract documents. This allows the contractor to understand, up front, his or her responsibilities regarding measure implementation. Any potential issues with implementation should be discussed and resolved before work begins.

SIDEBAR 4-1. Construction Specifications Institute Standardized Specification Divisions

Before the 1960s, standard specifications formats didn't exist. Each architectural, engineering, and contracting firm, as well as every government agency, had its own organizational system. That resulted in confusion and miscommunication among everyone involved in delivering construction projects, which led to costly delays, errors, and omissions. In 1962 the Construction Specifications Institute (CSI) developed the concept of divisions, and sections within each division, to standardize information in construction project manuals. Over the years, these divisions have evolved into a product that functions as the "Dewey Decimal System" for organizing specifications and other data. The most recent version of CSI's specifications includes 50 divisions that address traditional building specifications, as well as several rapidly developing areas such as telecommunications networks, integrated automation systems, and electronic safety and security systems. New sections have also been created to provide room for such things as more safety and security technology for buildings.[2] For more information about the 50 divisions, see the CSI Web site, www.csinet.org.

Conditions of the Contract

Conditions are written definitions of the responsibilities and interrelationships among parties involved in construction of the project as they pertain to the legal agreements between the organization and the contractor. These conditions reference general industry standards, building codes, and other requirements applicable to the project and contract documents. General conditions address generic issues pertinent to all construction projects. Supplementary conditions address issues specific to the construction project in question.

General Conditions. When creating a general conditions document, organizations may wish to consult the American Institute of Architects (AIA) document AIA's General Conditions of the Contract for Construction. This is a universally recognized model for general conditions that is thoroughly understood by design professionals, contractors, and construction lawyers alike.

Supplementary Conditions. The content of general conditions is broad and inclusive and cannot cover all aspects of a specific project. Supplementary conditions address specific project-related issues and facilitate modifications to general conditions. Examples of supplementary conditions include extensions of contract time due to changes in project scope, implementing ILSM and preconstruction risk assessment measures, and other issues. To ensure compliance with ILSM and preconstruction risk assessment measures, organizations may want to incorporate a mandatory adherence agreement into the construction contract. This should include penalties for noncompliance with ILSM and other measures.[3]

Construction Cost Estimate and Schedule

The construction documents phase completes the description of project construction content and supports a detailed construction budget. The size and quantity of significant building materials can be accurately estimated at this point in the process. Major equipment and special construction systems are also described and quantified, as are mechanical, electrical, and plumbing materials and systems. The quality level of significant materials and systems is defined. Construction budget contingencies can again be reduced to reflect the growing understanding of the project, and the allowance for inflation should be updated and refined at this point. Again, the project schedule requires updating.

Separate Contracts

An organization may elect to enter into separate contracts for designated portions of the project, especially for procurement and installation of expensive, highly specialized, technically sophisticated equipment. This is frequently done for data processing equipment, telecommunication systems, laboratory equipment, or radiological installations. These contracts should clearly identify the work as separately contracted and clarify its relationship to work in the prime construction contract.

Construction

The construction process is multifaceted and requires participation from all members of the project team, including organization leadership, staff, architects, engineers, contractors, and construction personnel. The specific responsibilities of each group will vary according to the size and scope of the project; however, generic activities must be performed in the construction phase of any project.

Beginning Construction

Before beginning construction, the project team should meet to discuss final preparations for construction. Within this meeting, participants should review project procedures, schedules, and budget; identify any necessary subcontractors; discuss plans to secure necessary building permits; determine actions for establishing project site security; and confirm that site conditions are acceptable for building the project as proposed. Other areas of discussion should include the following:

- Storage of building materials
- Contractors' access to occupied areas
- Relocation of furniture and equipment
- Above-ceiling access in occupied areas
- Barrier construction and placement
- Reaction plans for undesirable events
- Travel paths for contractors and deliveries
- Contractor education
- Contractor parking

Organizations may wish to consult the local fire marshal for any additional areas to discuss.

Before construction begins, the project team must implement relevant ILSM and measures that were developed as a response to the preconstruction risk assessment. Both the ILSM and preconstruction risk assessment should also be reviewed at this time to determine the emergence of new risks that need to be addressed.

Construction Worker Education

Although the general contractor should have health care experience, not all construction workers are familiar with the unique issues associated with a health care construction project. For example, a utility shutdown is something that must be carefully planned and coordinated in a health care facility. Workers can't just cut the power on a moment's notice or serious safety implications could arise. Some issues to cover in construction education include the following:

- Life safety risks and ILSM
- Infection control risks and measures to address those risks
- Security issues
- Parking and building access
- Patient privacy
- Proper waste handling
- Cell phone use
- Equipment and materials
- Radiation safety, if applicable
- Hazardous materials
- Utility/electrical safety
- Smoking
- Violence
- How to seek help and report issues

By including the ILSM and preconstruction risk assessment in the contract documents, the contractor can be aware of and educate construction workers on safety risks and preventive measures. The weekly construction meeting also provides opportunity for education. Some organizations require individual construction workers to receive training before they enter the construction site. This education might take the form of group training sessions or self-study guides. Contractors may keep a book that documents worker education so organizations can be assured that everyone received the proper education before coming on site. In smaller projects, the responsibility for construction worker education might fall to the facilities manager, safety manager, or infection control professional.

Communication During Construction

One of the most important components of the construction process is communication. Effective communication can mean the difference between a safe and successful project that is completed on time, and one that is plagued with delays, safety issues, budget overruns, and frustration. Organizations should ensure effective communication with and between the project team, organization staff, and patients.

The Project Team. Architects, engineers, contractors, and organization staff should all communicate frequently about the following issues:

- The status of the construction project
- The effectiveness of ILSM and other safety measures at preserving patient safety
- Any emerging safety concerns, such as infection control (IC) risks, fire safety risks, and so forth
- Any changes to the work
- Project budget
- Project schedule

Organizations may want to set up regular team meetings (some organizations choose to meet weekly) in which all issues are discussed. Issues that come up between meetings could be addressed via teleconference, videoconference, or e-mail. Representatives of the organization, along with the architect and consultants, should also visit the construction site on a regular basis during construction to become familiar with the progress of construction and to assist in determining whether the work is being conducted according to the contract documents. Organizations may wish to document these tours to monitor the progress of the project. IC and facilities management professionals should be a part of these construction tours to monitor ILSM, IC, and other safety measures.

Organization Staff and Patients. To prevent frustration, confusion, and risks to safety during a construction or renovation project, organizations must ensure effective communication with and between these two groups. Some things to communicate to staff and patients include the following:

- The nature of the construction project
- The time line involved
- What areas will be affected when
- How to safely enter and exit the building
- How to report safety risks observed during construction
- The precautions in place to preserve patient and staff safety, such as ILSM and IC measures
- New developments in the construction process

Organizations can use a variety of effective tools to communicate with staff and patients during the construction process. Following are a few such tools:

Staff training. Before construction begins, the organization may wish to conduct staff training sessions that describe the construction process and outline the responsibilities of staff members as they relate to that process. For example, IC professionals may want to educate staff on potential lapses in IC that staff should watch for and report. Facilities managers can inform staff of ILSM that are in place. By including staff as partners in the construction process, organizations can realize a safer experience for all.

Organization newsletter. An article in the organization's newsletter describing the project, time line, and general aspects of the initiative may be helpful to generate initial awareness among staff and patients. Updates as the project progresses can also be helpful.

Serial letter. Organization or project leaders may want to send a weekly letter to staff, numbered serially, that communicates the status of the project as of that week. The letter should outline what activities will happen during the week and describe the impact of those activities on staff. This letter could be sent via the mail, e-mail, or posted outside the construction site.

Web site. Many organizations create a dedicated Web site for the construction project. Patients and staff can access the site for information on the project scope, time line, and general updates.

Construction boards. Developed by Mel Trafford, M.A., C.H.F.M., C.F.P.S., director of facility management at St. Anthony Hospitals, a nonprofit multifacility health system centered in Denver, Colorado, construction boards inform staff, visitors, and anyone else coming into the facility of the existence and nature of a construction or renovation project. Construction boards are not required by the Joint Commission; however, they do provide an effective way to give individuals information about safety and other important topics. They can be a good way to handle communication about general safety rules, and they can alert hospital staff, contractors, patients, family members, and others to important changes in the construction process. (*See* Sidebar 4-2, on pages 108–109.)

The Public. In addition to staff and patients, organizations should communicate with the public about the nature, time line, and projected outcomes of a construction project. Depending on the particular construction project, the public may be significantly affected by such issues as altered traffic patterns and increased noise levels. By taking a proactive approach to communication, organizations can prevent miscommunication and confusion that could lead to an adverse relationship between the organization and the public.

Information about a construction or renovation project can be disseminated through a variety of venues, including press releases, commercials, public announcements, organization newsletters, and the organization Web site.

Implementing and Monitoring ILSM and Other Safety Measures

Chapter Three discussed ILSM and proactive risk assessment. Several other aspects of those processes must occur as the organization begins construction. These aspects include the following:

Implement identified measures. As previously mentioned, some of these measures may include barriers, signage, high-efficiency particulate air (HEPA) filtered fans and vacuums, clean and dirty rooms, specific traffic patterns, negative pressure rooms, and environmental monitoring. (*See* Sidebar 4-3 on page 110.) Contractors should be involved in the implementation process. Many times contractors will be in charge of implementation, but organizations should verify that this implementation does, in fact, occur.

Post measures. This could include posting via posters and construction boards placed near the entrance to the construction site. Organizations that have a project Web site should also consider posting measures on that site.

Educate construction workers. As previously mentioned, the contractor may be in charge of this effort, but organizations should reinforce education during weekly construction meetings.

Educate staff. This could involve training staff members on any identified safety risks; on measures to address those risks, including ILSM and infection control measures; and on how to report activities that occur without the proper risk prevention measures.

Case Study 4-1, beginning on page 110, illustrates how two organizations implemented ILSM, IC, and other safety measures during construction.

Stopping Work. During regular construction site visits or based on reports from staff, organization leaders, facility managers, IC professionals, and safety officers may learn of a hazardous condition that needs prompt attention. These individuals should be given authority to stop all work until the issue is addressed, if that is warranted. In addition, the person or persons responsible for air and water quality monitoring must be given authority to stop the construction work if a problem develops.

Cleaning Up

Organizations should make sure that the construction team takes adequate steps to clean the site throughout construction. The time to establish cleaning agreements is, of course, before construction begins. Too many stories exist of soda cans and cigarette butts being sealed in walls because of inadequate clean up. These items can lead to mold, fungi, and bacteria issues.

During construction, the contractor can keep the construction area clean by taking the following actions:

- Having staging areas properly allocated for materials being delivered to and being stored on the site
- Keeping absorbent materials protected from moisture
- Suppressing dust with wetting agents or sweeping compounds
- Cleaning up immediately after activities that produce high dust levels, or at the end of each day the activity continues

SIDEBAR 4-2. Construction Boards

Construction boards offer a comprehensive method for communicating with staff and patients about a construction project. According to Mel Trafford of St. Anthony Hospitals in Denver, construction boards are simple to build. Following are the six steps involved:

1. Start with a piece of 1/4-inch plywood measuring approximately 24 inches high by 46 inches wide.
2. Add a 3/4-inch wooden border around the edge.
3. Attach a 5/8-inch vertical divider in the middle of the board to create two equal display sections.
4. One section is for more-or-less permanent *general* information. Cover this section with a piece of 1/8-inch Plexiglas (attach with wing nuts).
5. The other section is for *specific* information that changes frequently. Cover this side with a thin layer of cork.
6. Before the start of a project, place one board—sitting on a tripod—at each entrance to the work site. Normally, only one or two boards are required.

"The board's general information section," says Trafford, "should feature things like work permits and project time lines." This section should also include important safety information, such as the following:

- ILSM in place for the duration of the project
- Fire safety policies, including alarm codes and information on fire classes
- Fire safety procedures, including RACE (rescue-alarm-confine-extinguish) and PASS (pull-aim-squeeze-sweep)
- Emergency evacuation routes
- Locations of fire extinguishers
- Infection control and air quality information

Trafford says the specific information section is for communications that may change monthly, weekly, or daily, such as project updates and schedule information. It is also the place to post safety-related information, including the following:

- Updates and changes to ILSM procedures
- Infection control checklists
- Noise abatement notifications

To convey information about construction noise, Trafford has developed a special "sound scale" similar to the "pain scale" clinicians use (*see* Sidebar 4-2a on page 109). Sound scale information changes every day, with updates on what noise level to expect at what hour.

When using construction boards, Trafford recommends keeping language issues in mind. Key information should be translated into any foreign language spoken by a large part of the community. In addition, illustrations and international symbols should be used whenever possible.

Link to Many Audiences

"The construction board addresses so many different things in a concentrated area," states Trafford. "It's a good method of communication—and a teaching tool." Construction boards can allow health care facilities to fulfill ILSM requirements for fire safety, especially with respect to alternative exits, additional fire-fighting equipment, and temporary deficiencies such as impaired compartmentalization features. The boards can also be used to reinforce the prohibition against smoking. They are particularly useful for conveying safety information and other hospital policies to contractors.

According to Trafford, construction boards also promote cooperation between construction crews and hospital staff. Construction noise provides a good example. Above a certain level, work noise can drown out patient monitor alarms. It can interrupt routine clinical tasks, such as taking vital signs, and also be a serious disruption during surgery. Sound scale notices on the construction board open a dialogue between the construction crew and hospital staff. Nurses get a chance to express their concerns, which gives contractors the chance to work out alternatives. "It gives nurses input and control," says Trafford.

Continued on page 109

SIDEBAR 4-2. Construction Boards, continued

He also noted that construction boards are useful in communicating with physicians. Many physicians work at three or four different hospitals, each of which may be undergoing several construction projects at any given time. Construction boards give physicians the information they need, when and where they need it.

The information boards also foster good working relationships with inspectors. "When fire marshals come in, they love seeing the boards," Trafford states. "It shows them we are working with safety issues." Infection control inspectors are also appreciative.

Trafford advocates using digital photography to document IC compliance. "Digital imagery allows us to replace written checklists," he says. "Pictures can serve as proof-positive to any compliance officer that certain measures were in place at the onset and inspected throughout the project." Trafford notes that posting photos on the construction board lets hospital staff and others support the compliance effort. For example, if a photo shows a closed door sealed with tape, and a nurse sees that the door is open, the nurse can inform workers immediately.

Construction Boards Provide a Way to Link with Patients and Visitors

"Normally, construction areas are walled off," says Trafford. Construction boards with photo documentation let visitors see the large number of protective measures in place. "In some respects, the board tells patients we are concerned," he says. "It's a little bit of a marketing tool for our commitment to patient safety."

Never Too Much

Trafford believes construction boards are an effective way to share information—and sharing information is essential to overcoming the challenges of health care construction. "In the hospital industry, renovation and new construction are daily events," he says. "You can never communicate enough on a construction project."

SIDEBAR 4-2A. Sound Scale

Trafford developed a special "sound scale" that helps hospital staff plan for disruptions caused by construction noise. The scale defines noise levels in terms staff members can easily understand (*see* below). Daily notices (posted on construction boards) let staff know what noise level to expect at what hour. Clinicians can work around expected noise interruptions or, if need be, ask construction crews to reschedule particularly disruptive activities. "The scale helps people associate the noise level with the type of construction or demolition," Trafford says. He notes that hospitals can use any numbering system or set of examples to create a sound scale. "The best thing to do is work with your safety committee to come up with definitions your staff will understand."

Sound Scale
Level Examples and Equivalents

1
Normal talking

2
Steady hammering
Alarm clock
Police whistle

3
Drilling
Home lawn mower
Truck with no muffler

4
Circular saw
Shot hammer
Car horn at 10 feet

5
Jackhammer
Cement cutter

- Replacing any absorbent materials that become exposed to moisture during construction
- Vacuuming stud tracks prior to application of second surface of gypsum board, to remove dirt and potential food sources for mold
- Keeping duct ends sealed with plastic to reduce dust infiltration into the mechanical system when the system is not in use
- Covering return air registers with filter material if the mechanical system must be used during construction

Some things organizations should require of construction teams at the end of construction include the following:

- Area is cleared, cleaned, and decontaminated
- Work area is vacuumed with HEPA–filtered vacuums
- Area is mopped with disinfectant
- Barriers are removed with care to minimize the spread of dust and debris. Above-mentioned cleaning should occur after barriers are removed
- Barriers should be disposed of properly
- Construction waste is bagged or transported in covered carts
- Air vents are unblocked

SIDEBAR 4-3. Air and Water Testing

If a construction project requires frequent air and water testing, it is important to have this testing done by someone who is qualified to perform such testing. Although a larger organization may have a certified industrial hygienist on staff, a smaller organization may need to bring in someone.

Staff should define culturing or sampling procedures before beginning work and establish parameters for interpreting collected data. Performing as much real-time monitoring as possible is important.

"Instruments that indicate right away whether there's a problem (as opposed to testing methods that require sending samples to laboratories and waiting for results) let you address the problem immediately," notes David C. Regelbrugge, C.I.H., C.S.P., senior safety and health consultant with Aires Consulting Group in Batavia, Illinois.

Case Study 4-1. Implementing and Monitoring Life Safety and Infection Control Risks

Two Organizations Take a Comprehensive Approach to Addressing Safety Risks in Construction

Although assessing safety risks associated with construction is very important, the assessment process will mean nothing if control measures to address identified risks are not implemented and monitored for success. In addition, the construction process will more than likely lead to the emergence of further safety risks, and organizations should vigilantly monitor these risks.

Both Elmhurst Memorial Healthcare and St. Alphonsus Regional Medical Center work diligently to ensure implementation of control measures and monitoring of emergent risks.

Elmhurst Memorial Healthcare

Just before construction begins at Elmhurst Memorial Healthcare in Elmhurst, Illinois, a list of control measures is posted at all entrances to the construction site. The organization developed standardized forms to use as ILSM, infection control risk assessment, and general construction disruption posting sheets. Elmhurst Memorial Healthcare color coded these forms. (*See* Figures 4-2, 4-3, and 4-4 on pages 111–113 for examples of these posting sheets.) The posting sheets require the name of the project, start date, completion date, location of the project, and the measures implemented. The posting sheets are designed to be easy to read and understand, so that staff, patients, and construction personnel can easily understand the control measures in place. The posting sheet lists a phone number for staff to use to report issues. "We rely on staff to help ensure ILSM and infection control compliance. It involves them in the safety process and also serves as a double check for the facilities, security, and infection control departments," says Dave Samples, facilities engineer for Elmhurst Memorial Healthcare.

Continued on page 111

Continued from page 110

FIGURE 4-2 ILSM Posting Sheet

ATTENTION
THIS AREA UNDER INTERIM LIFE SAFETY MEASURES

Due to construction project work, this entire area is under temporary interim life safety measures (ILSM) and surveillance until completion of all work. Any failure to comply with any of these measures should be reported to Safety & Protection at 41500 immediately

Name of Project ____________________

Start Date ____________ Completion Date ____________

Area of Project ____________________

Areas Under ILSM ____________________

MEASURES IMPLEMENTED

❏ Firewatch required

❏ Hourly watch ❏ Daily watch ❏ Permanent watch

❏ Daily Hazard Surveillance (@3 PM)

❏ Department Education on____________ ❏ Double Fire drills

❏ Exit Impact?____________

❏ Daily cleaning up of all combustable materials & trash

❏ One hour fire/smoke partitions?____________

❏ All penetrations in fire/smoke walls sealed?

❏ All fire detection/suppression systems operational

❏ Fire extinguishers present and not blocked

Elmhurst Memorial Healthcare developed this standardized posting sheet to educate staff and patients on the ILSM aspects of the construction project.

Source: Elmhurst Memorial Healthcare, Elmhurst, IL.

To deal with the possibility of general construction disruptions such as noise, vibration, and the like, Samples also uses posting sheets. Before a project begins, Samples posts notices at all areas that are overhead of, underneath, and adjacent to the work areas. Staff in the affected areas are informed of the upcoming work, and the notices on the walls give them a means of directly contacting the work site in order to minimize the disturbances both to the medical staffs and the patients and family members. One phone call will connect the staff with the work area in order to temporarily stop or postpone the construction in order to work around patient care. Not only do concerns all go through an organization stop, the staff are also happy to know about the work ahead of time. "An added benefit," says Samples, "is that most staff will also call and tell us when a patient is gone for an MRI, a surgical case is finished, or a physician has gone to lunch so that work can resume ASAP without irritating anyone."

At the beginning of a project, Elmhurst's infection control practitioner meets with staff and managers to educate them on IC measures. In addition, the organization requires the contractor to educate all construction workers on safety issues and prevention measures. Because Elmhurst includes the ILSM and IC control measures in the bid package, the contractor is familiar with the education

Continued on page 112

Continued from page 111

FIGURE 4-3 Infection Control Posting Sheet

ATTENTION
THIS AREA UNDER CONSTRUCTION
INFECTION CONTROL MEASURES

Due to construction project work, this entire area is under temporary "Construction Infection Control Measures and Surveillance" until completion of all work. Any failure to comply with any of these measures should be reported to the Infection Control Practitioner immediately at Ext. 41414 or Pgr. XXX-XXX-XXXX

Name of Project: ____________________
Start Date: ____________________ Completion Date: ____________________

MEASURES IMPLEMENTED
❑ Portable HEPA Filteration Unit
❑ Negative Pressure
❑ Outside Exhaust
❑ Temporary Walls (slab to slab and airtight)
❑ Plastic Sheeting (airtight)
❑ Sticky Entrance Mats and Entrances
❑ Daily HEPA Vacuuming
❑ Daily Wet Mopping
❑ All Supply & Return Vents Sealed Off
❑ Daily Removal of Trash & Broom Clean
❑ Closing of All Doors to Patient Care Areas

INFECTION CONTROL EVALUATION SCORE = ____________

Elmhurst Memorial Healthcare developed this standardized posting sheet to educate staff and patients on the infection control aspects of the construction project.

Source: Elmhurst Memorial Healthcare, Elmhurst, IL.

that is necessary. Additional training is provided during weekly construction meetings. "We include the infection control practitioner in weekly construction team meetings. This helps continue focus on infection control issues throughout construction," Samples says.

As construction proceeds, the facilities management and security staff monitor the construction site for compliance with safety and infection control measures. An IC practitioner regularly checks for compliance as well. Should any one of these individuals identify a safety issue, he or she has the authority to stop the project until the issue is corrected.

Although the contractor is required to implement most measures, the organization did buy two HEPA filtration units to be used during construction projects. "Not only does this ensure proper air filtration during projects, but we manage the maintenance and cleaning of these units and can, therefore, ensure the use of proper maintenance and cleaning procedures," Samples notes.

St. Alphonsus Regional Medical Center

During construction projects at St. Alphonsus in Boise, Idaho, the contractor, IC practitioner, security officer, safety officer, and facilities manager have a weekly meeting to discuss project issues,

Continued on page 113

Continued from page 112

FIGURE 4-4 Construction Disruption Posting Sheet

ATTENTION
THIS AREA TO EXPERIENCE
CONSTRUCTION DISRUPTIONS

DUE TO CONSTRUCTION WORK IN THE IMMEDIATE VICINITY, THIS AREA IS EXPECTED TO EXPERIENCE WORK-RELATED DISRUPTIONS, INCLUDING NOISE, DUST, INCREASED TRAFFIC, VIBRATIONS, DRILLING, & INTERRUPTIONS OF WORK AND/OR UTILITIES. EVERY EFFORT WILL BE MADE TO MINIMIZE THE DISTURBANCES, & ALL WORK WILL BE COORDINATED TO REDUCE THE IMPACT ON OPERATIONS

Name of Project: ______________________________

Area of Construction Work: ______________________________

Adjacent Areas Affected by Work: ______________________________

Start Date: ______________ Completion Date: ______________

Name of Construction Contractor: ______________________________

Construction Site Phone Number: ______________________

Emergency Contractor Number: ______________________

Project Manager: ______________________________

If in the event of an emergency, unplanned loss of utilities, or emergency work stoppage request, please contact the following numbers in order:

1.) David Samples—Facilities Engineer—ext. 44888/pgr. 1523
2.) Facilities Management 24-Hour Service—ext. 44444
3.) Security & Protection—ext. 41500/pgr. 0101

Elmhurst Memorial Healthcare developed this standardized posting sheet to inform staff and patients that the construction project is taking place and to give staff a way to contact the construction authorities.

Source: Elmhurst Memorial Healthcare, Elmhurst, IL.

new developments, and so forth. After this meeting, the group walks through the construction site to verify implementation of ILSM and IC measures, as well as to identify any emerging hazards. St. Alphonsus uses a surveillance form to verify that required ILSM are in place. (*See* Figure 4-5 on page 114.)

"Although we do conduct the life safety and infection control assessments separately, monitoring compliance with control measures is a team process. The contractor, infection control practitioner, security office, safety officer, and facilities manager are all watching out for infection control and life safety issues and making sure any required control measures are implemented," says William Morgan, manager of plant operations and facility engineering for St. Alphonsus.

St. Alphonsus requires all construction personnel to receive training, before they start work, on such topics as the IC, life safety, and security issues associated with the construction project. "We don't issue a name badge until a construction worker can prove he or she has been trained on the issues associated with the project," Morgan says. "Our safety and security department devel-

Continued on page 114

FIGURE 4-5 ILSM Hazard Surveillance

ILSM Hazard Surveillance

Project: Coordinator: Start Date / / End Date: / / Inspector:

Description of work:

Notes:

Initials of person doing check	Check if Required																															
Chart by: Days ____ Hours ____ For: Month ____ Year ____		1	2	3	4	5	6	7	8	9	10	11	12	13	14	15	16	17	18	19	20	21	22	23	24	25	26	27	28	29	30	31
1. Free/unobstructed exits. Egress routes clear.																																
2. Corridors clear of obstruction.																																
3. Emergency exits unobstructed.																																
4. Temporary partitions in place and smoke tight.																																
5. Construction site clean and orderly.																																
6. Alternate routes for public access.																																
7. Pull boxes unobstructed.																																
8. Warning signage clear.																																
9. Fire protection systems functioning.																																
10. Fire extinguishers/hoses unobstructed.																																
11. Fire doors unobstructed.																																
12. Staff educated on deficiencies.																																
13. Hazardous materials stored properly.																																

St. Alophonsus uses this form to verify that ILSM are in place.

Source: St. Alphonsus Regional Medical Center, Boise, ID.

Continued on page 115

Continued from page 114

oped a training program and, depending on the size of the project, the facility manager, infection control practitioner, or the contractor may be in charge of training efforts."

In both organizations, the safety assessment and control measure implementation processes are continuous throughout the life of the construction project. "Depending on the size of the project, we may conduct more than one assessment. Each phase—site preparation, demolition, and construction—may have its own assessment and control measures," notes Morgan.

By frequently walking through the construction site, listening to reports of staff, and regularly communicating with contractors, both organizations can ensure a continuous emphasis on safety during construction.

CASE AT A GLANCE

■ **Main challenge**
To implement ILSM, IC, and other safety measures. To continuously monitor the construction site for emerging risks.

■ **Issues**
Implementation is typically done by the contractor; however, organizations must continuously ensure that all measures are in place and effective.

■ **Solutions**
Both organizations regularly tour the construction site and solicit help from the staff to monitor safety issues.

■ **Outcomes**
By frequently revisiting the preconstruction risk assessment and ILSM assessment, the two organizations can identify issues early and implement measures to address those issues.

REFERENCES

1. Reiling J., et al.: Enhancing the traditional hospital design process: A focus on patient safety. *Joint Commission Journal on Quality and Safety* 30:115–124, Mar. 2004.

2. Construction Specifications Institute: *About Master Format 2004 Edition.* Construction Specifications Institute. http://www.csinet.org/s_csi/sec.asp?TRACKID=&CID=852&DID=10076 (accessed Aug. 15, 2005).

3. Old L.: Construction risk management. Paper presented at the ASHE International Conference and Exhibition on Health Facility Planning Design and Construction, Chicago, Mar. 7, 2005.

CHAPTER FIVE:

Commissioning

BUILDING COMMISSIONING ensures that building systems operate efficiently, meet the needs of the organization, function as designed, and maintain the comfort of occupants.[1] In addition, organizations must answer the following questions during the commissioning process:

- Does the building reflect the design agreed upon by the organization?
- Are all changes to the design that were made since construction documents were drawn and were agreed to by the organization reflected in the building?
- Is the content of the building correct? In other words, is the equipment, furniture, wall coverings, floor coverings, fixtures, electrical outlets, lights, and so forth what the organization agreed to?
- Does everything work the way it should?
- Is everything compliant with all applicable regulations and laws?

Commissioning has been compared to test driving a car; however, it is much more than that. It is akin to asking not only if the car works, but if all the components of the car are present. In some ways, the commissioning process is like the final walk-through of a newly constructed home, except on a much larger scale. New homeowners verify every aspect of their new abode, as health care organizations will do with their newly constructed facility.

Building commissioning should be a systematic process that involves verifying and documenting that all building systems and features are present and perform interactively according to the intent of the design and the organization's needs. The process should begin in the design phase and may last at least one year after the project is finished. Key elements in building commissioning include the following:

- Thoroughly documenting system design intent, operating sequences, and test procedures
- Verifying system performance based on extensive functional testing and measurement
- Training building operations staff on system operation and maintenance procedures
- Ongoing monitoring of system performance[1]

Although the concept of commissioning is not challenging, the implementation can be very difficult. Consider a newly constructed 100-bed nursing unit that needs to be commissioned. Those in charge of commissioning must verify all aspects of every room, hallway, bathroom, break room, nurses' station, boiler room, and so forth. For large projects, the commissioning process can be quite daunting.

Who Is in Charge of Commissioning?

Depending on the type and scope of the project, as well as the organization's preferences, one of three parties can be responsible for commissioning:

Organization representatives. A facility manager or the project leader may be an appropriate choice for commissioning, depending on the project. Organizations may want to consider developing a multidisciplinary team for commissioning. This will ensure that important aspects of design are not overlooked. Members of the team may include the following:

- Facility manager
- Safety manager
- Infection control professional
- Facilities engineers and representatives from the maintenance team
- Representative from the area under construction, such as a nurse manager, pharmacy manager, laboratory manger, and so forth
- Organization leader

Representatives of the organization are familiar with the project as well as the organization's goals for the project. Because of this, they have unique insight into the commissioning process. However, the commissioning process may be too much for one person or a small group of people to handle, particularly people who do not have a lot of experience in commissioning. Organization representatives may overlook issues or find it difficult to combine commissioning efforts with their regular duties.

The contractor. The contractor is also familiar with the project and can easily determine if things are working well or not. Organizations that choose to have their contractor spearhead the commissioning process must have a lot of faith and trust in the contractor and feel confident that the contractor will not misrepresent the status of the building.

A third party that is hired by the organization or the contractor. This person is typically called the commissioning agent. Those involved in the building commissioning field generally believe that the commissioning agent should work for the owner and represent the owner's interest. However, numerous options exist. The commissioning agent can work under contract to the construction manager. This works well when the construction manager is independent of the contractor's team. Several architect and engineering firms are interested in including commissioning as part of their services to ensure that they deliver quality buildings to their clients.[1] Of all the parties that could spearhead the commissioning process, a commissioning agent would probably have the most expertise and could streamline the process. The commissioning agent can also offer a fresh perspective. However, third-party contractors do cost money, and if the building project is over budget, spending further funds for commissioning efforts may not be feasible.

When deciding who should commission a building, organizations should keep in mind the needs of the organization, the nature of the project, the budget involved with the project, and the time allowed for commissioning.

Before embarking on the process, organizations may want to research different professional organizations' recommendations for commissioning. For example, the American Society of Heating, Refrigeration, and Air-Conditioning Engineers offers some specific guidelines for the commissioning process.

How It Works

The commissioning process can vary by project. Ideally, it begins during predesign and continues after the acceptance of the building. During predesign, the organization should establish the parameters and expectations of commissioning. During design, the following issues related to commissioning should be outlined:

- Design intent
- The systems to be installed
- Documentation requirements for each party involved in the commissioning process

Typically, the commissioning plan is completed at the beginning of the construction phase. Project schedules, as well as contractor documents and operation and maintenance manuals, are reviewed. A detailed performance test plan should be written for each system and piece of equipment involved in the commissioning process. Any construction details that might affect equipment and system performance or operation should be noted. Whoever is doing the commissioning should coordinate with the various contractors to perform the prefunctional performance tests during construction.

In addition to developing system and equipment test plans, the individual or team in charge of commissioning should verify that the following items are present and meet the organization's expectations:

- Power plant issues (pumps, deaeration tanks, softeners, and so forth.)
- Heating, ventilating, and air-conditioning (HVAC) equipment
- Water distribution and plumbing
- Electrical distribution (switch boards, main circuit boards, bus bars, and so forth)
- Finishes
- Flooring
- Standardization
- Life safety features and compliance, such as fire alarms, sprinklers, smoke barriers, fire doors, and so forth
- Furniture
- Windows and window treatments
- Doors and door locks
- Outlets
- Communication systems
- Computer systems
- Signage
- Wall coverings
- Ceiling tiles
- Paving
- Landscaping
- Roofs
- Insulation
- Elevators
- Infection control (*see* Sidebar 5-1 on page 120)
- Other

Before the building is accepted, the individual or individuals in charge of commissioning should observe and verify the proper operation of equipment, systems, and controls per contract documents (*see* Sidebar 5-2 on page 121). Any corrective actions must be verified, and complete operation and maintenance manuals should be present. Actual performance testing is typically carried out by the various contractors. After all performance tests are complete, the individual or team in charge of commissioning should issue a final report, including all documentation.[1]

Making the Process Manageable

Some organizations use a checklist to organize the commissioning process and ensure that all aspects of building design, construction, and content are verified. Organizations may want to use the 50 material and building system specification sections developed by the Construction Specifications Institute (*see* Chapter Four, page 104) as a framework for the checklist. Organizations must customize the checklist for the particular construction project and include information from construction documents and any changes made during construction.

Creating this checklist will take time, but can help manage the commissioning process.

Organizations that start creating the checklist when construction documents are finalized can ensure that all aspects of the project are contained in the checklist.

Allow Time for Commissioning

Effective commissioning cannot be done overnight. For some projects, it can begin up to six months prior to the turnover of the building. Operational components of the building, such as equipment, boilers, and HVAC equipment, can be tested while construction is under way and, in fact, often are commissioned right at the original equipment manufacturers' factory. If a component will not change before the building is occupied, it can be commissioned early. For example, after equipment such as radiology or laboratory equipment has been installed, the individuals in charge of commissioning can verify the presence of the equipment and ensure that it works. Starting the commissioning process early, and allowing plenty of time for it, can reduce the stress involved and prevent those in charge of commissioning from getting overwhelmed.

Punch List

As an organization goes through the commissioning process, the organization's representative, in conjunction with the design team, should create a punch list. This is a list of all the things that need to be addressed in the building before occupancy. Issues such as equipment that does not function correctly, an incorrect wall finish in the surgical suites, inappropriate door handles in isolation rooms, and so forth are things that could go on a punch list. The contractor is required to correct all issues on a punch list before the organization accepts the building.

The punch list should be started during construction. Many things need to be caught early so that they are not concealed in the construction or duplicated unnecessarily. Items for the punch list should be noted during field observations by the architect, engineer, organization representative, or commissioning agent throughout the construction process.

In addition to the organization's punch list, the contractor should always complete a punch list and correct any deficiencies found. This ensures that the contractor presents the most complete work for review.

Although the punch list can be started during construction, a final punch list is created just prior to building acceptance. This punch list is developed during the final walk-through of the building and hopefully contain relatively minor issues that need attention.

SIDEBAR 5-1.
Infection Control Issues

Some important infection control (IC) questions to answer during commissioning include the following:

- Are sinks properly located and functioning?
- Do sinks in critical patient care areas have properly functioning fixtures?
- Are aerators present or absent in these fixtures, according to facility policy?
- Are soap and towel dispensers filled and functioning?
- Are surfaces in procedure and service areas appropriate for use? (For example, are they smooth, nonporous, and water resistant?)
- Has air balancing been completed according to specifications?
- Does air flow into negative pressure rooms and out of positive pressure rooms?[2]

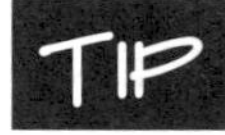

Using a Punch List to Assess *Life Safety Code*® Compliance

As previously mentioned, assessing *Life Safety Code*®* (*LSC*) compliance is one area of the commissioning process. Any areas of noncompliance should be reflected on the punch list. Because a life safety analysis looks at the same issues that the commissioning process does, organizations can use the commissioning process and punch list to assess *LSC* compliance and report areas of noncompliance. ■

Documenting the Process

To prevent duplication of efforts or omission of important aspects of the building from commissioning, organizations should document the commissioning process. This may include creating a database

* *Life Safety Code*® is a registered trademark of the National Fire Protection Association, Quincy, MA.

that houses information on areas of acceptance as well as items for the punch list. Project staff may want to periodically review this database during commissioning to keep abreast of punch list issues and their resolutions.

Budgeting for Commissioning

Commissioning not only involves a monetary cost (hiring a third-party commissioner or paying the contractor for commissioning efforts), it also involves a time cost. If an organization chooses to have organization representatives do the commissioning, those representatives must be allowed time in their schedules to effectively perform commissioning tasks. This may require temporarily reassigning their regular job duties to someone else.

Organizations should budget both the time and monetary aspects of commissioning upfront in the project budget so costs do not come as a surprise at the end of the construction process.

Occupancy

As organizations prepare to take occupancy, plans should be developed for moving and employee orientation. Organizations may also want to revisit some of their policies. A new facility can be an opportune time to introduce new procedures, protocols, and ways of conducting day-to-day activities.

Training for the building operation staff generally occurs around the time of occupancy. The training should be done by the installing contractors, designers, and manufacturers' representatives and may include any third-party commissioning agents.[1]

Organizations may want to use the commissioning process as a time to train staff on the content, layout, and design of the building. Training staff on the building before occupancy ensures the staff are familiar with the content and operation of the building from day one. This can minimize disruptions in patient care as staff members familiarize themselves with equipment, room layout, and supply location.

After the final walk-through has taken place and most items on the punch list have been addressed (often, minor punch list items are still open at this time), the city, county, and state will come on site and take a final walk-through of the building. After these entities give their blessing, the contractor turns over the building to the organization for occupancy. This is a time for celebration. In most cases, the planning, design, and construction process will have taken many years to complete. Organizations should celebrate their success and acknowledge the work of the staff involved in the project. While some staff members will have dedicated great time and effort to the process, all staff will be involved in some way. Celebrations should acknowledge the participation of everyone in the planning, design, and construction process. It is a team effort, the impact of which will be felt for years to come.

SIDEBAR 5-2. Systems Commissioning

During systems commissioning consider taking the following important steps:

- Owner review the table of contents of operating and maintaining (O&M) manuals at beginning of construction
- Use a close-out log
- Provide all close-out submittals at substantial completion
- Photograph installations
- Record drawings based on contractor marked-up as-built drawings, prepared by design team
- Summarize all warranty contact information in one section of O&M manual
- In-service owner as equipment is contractor tested
- Coordinate designer participation
- Perform air testing after all ceilings are installed
- Review fire and smoke wall systems with owner as work is installed
- Provide test/certification data as soon as possible
- Videotape all major equipment in-service sessions

REFERENCES

1. Western Area Power Administration, WSUEEP98018, Rev. 2/98. Funded by the National Institute of Building Sciences (NIBS): *Building Commissioning for New Construction.* http://www.betterbricks.com/default.aspx?pid=article&articleid=155&typeid=8&topicname=commissioning&indextype=topic (accessed Aug. 15, 2005).

2. Bartley J.: APIC state-of-the-art report: The role of infection control during construction in health care facilities. *Am J Infect Control* 28:156–159, 2000.

APPENDIX A:

Special Considerations for the Design of Laboratories

DEPENDING ON THE NATURE of the construction project, organizations may need to design and build a laboratory. Most of this publication has addressed considerations for patient care rooms and support rooms. Because of the nature of the work provided in laboratories, there are some special considerations that organizations should keep in mind during planning, design, and construction. Some of these considerations include the following:

- Safety
- Ventilation
- Storage
- Acoustics

Safety and Security

As with other areas of the health care facility, safety and security are paramount when designing laboratories. There has been a lot of concern about bioterrorism and the threats to safety that can be realized through terrorist activity. The reality is that laboratory scientists deal with biohazardous materials every day, and some of these materials can be equally as harmful as any potential bioterrorist weapons. It is incumbent on organization management to protect their staff and the surrounding environment from exposure to biohazardous material, no matter what its origins.

Before planning for a laboratory project, laboratory and organization management should determine the laboratory's potential biohazard level and design and equip the laboratory to contain hazardous materials appropriate to that level. The Centers for Disease Control and Prevention (CDC) identifies four biosafety levels for laboratories that help organizations categorize their risks and determine what controls should be in place to appropriately contain those risks (*see* Sidebar A-1 on page 125).

Different safety precautions will be necessary depending on the biosafety designation of the lab. The scope of this publication does not allow in-depth discussion of each possible safety feature; however, following is a brief discussion on some of the more common safety controls.

A negatively pressurized area. As discussed in Chapters Three and Four, negatively pressurized areas are critical to prevent the spread of airborne contaminants. The laboratory should be a negatively pressurized area to prevent contaminants from escaping into the rest of the facility.

Biosafety cabinets and hoods. These units can provide a cleaner work environment, protect laboratory staff against aerosols, and contain the spread of infectious agents. The number and classification of these hoods will depend on the laboratory's assessed biosafety level and the specific procedures the hoods are being used for. "It is especially important to locate biosafety cabinets away from doors, air supply fans, drafts, and heavily trafficked areas. Disruptions in adjacent air flow dramatically limit the effectiveness of biosafety cabinets," says Karen Mortland, American Institute of Architects (AIA), M.T. (ASCP), president of Mortland Planning and Design.

Completely cleanable spaces. Carpets should never be used in the laboratory, and any floor, wall, or counter spaces should be completely cleanable. Epoxy paint should be used, when possible, and coved surfaces are recommended to prevent the pooling of infectious material. In addition, strong bleach solutions can cause corrosion on stainless steel countertops, making chemically resistant plastic laminate or epoxy resin counters the preferred materials for this use.[1]

Hands-free hand-wash sinks. Because of the nature of the work in the laboratory, these type of sinks can minimize the spread of hazardous materials. Laboratory personnel can decontaminate their hands without contaminating sink faucets.

Magnetic hold-opens. Doors between adjacent laboratory areas traveled by laboratory personnel should be on a magnetic hold-open tied to the fire alarm system. However, doors that are used for separations from public areas or for pressurization changes should never be kept open. For security reasons access doors to the laboratory should be locked so entrance to the lab can be restricted and monitored.

Emergency showers and eyewash stations. The American National Standards Institute (ANSI), the CDC, and the Americans with Disabilities Act (ADA) all have requirements about the proper design, location, and signage for emergency showers and eyewash stations. For example, ANSI requires eyewash stations to be easily accessible. Staff should be able to reach an eyewash station in no more than 10 seconds, if necessary. The sinks should be within a travel distance of 100 feet from the hazard. Architects, engineers, and laboratory managers should be familiar with the requirements surrounding this equipment and address these requirements during design and construction.

Ventilation

Because of new technology that takes up more room and the trend toward consolidating labs within a facility, many health care organization laboratories are crowded with equipment and people. (Also, in

SIDEBAR A-1. Biosafety Levels

Laboratory biosafety levels fall into four classifications. Each successive level includes and expands on the requirements of the preceding one.

Biosafety Level One

Biosafety level one (BSL-1) is the designation for labs handling agents not known to consistently cause disease in healthy adult humans. Such labs do not have to be separated from general traffic patterns, but doors are required and access to the lab should be limited or restricted at the discretion of laboratory management when work is in progress. BSL-1 labs must be equipped with a hand-wash sink, and all surfaces must be easily cleaned. Carpets and rugs are not permitted. Eating, drinking, smoking, handling contact lenses, applying cosmetics, and storing food is not permitted.

Biosafety Level Two

Biosafety level two (BSL-2) labs may handle agents of moderate potential hazard. With the exceptions of culturing some virology, some mycology, and tuberculosis, as well as some molecular testing, most clinical lab areas fall into this classification. This is because of the potential presence of bloodborne pathogens, such as tuberculosis and HIV, in any clinical specimen. In addition to BSL-1 requirements, BSL-2 labs should be located away from public areas and be fitted with lockable doors. A hand-wash sink and eyewash station should be readily available. Airflow design should be negative, pulling air away from doorways and preventing aerosols from escaping the lab. No air should recirculate to any spaces outside the laboratory.

Biosafety Level Three

Biosafety level three (BSL-3) labs work with indigenous or exotic agents that can cause serious or potentially lethal disease. The clinical lab exceptions mentioned above fall under BSL-3 requirements. Most bioterrorism agents may be safely handled in BSL-3 areas with the exceptions of smallpox and viral hemorrhagic fevers, which should be confined to BSL-4 labs. BSL-3 labs must be separated from other parts of the building by an anteroom with two sets of self-closing doors or by access through a BSL-2 area. Doors must be lockable and, optionally, a clothes changing room may be included in the passageway. A hands-free or automatic hand-wash sink and an emergency eyewash station must be located near the room exit. Procedures involving the manipulation of infectious materials must be done in a biosafety cabinet or other physical containment device. Therefore, a biosafety cabinet is required in BSL-3 labs and must be properly located.

Solid floors and ceilings are required with all penetrations sealed. Construction materials must be smooth, impermeable to liquids, and resistant to chemicals and disinfectants normally used in the lab. Gypsum or plaster painted with epoxy paint is acceptable for ceilings. Floors should be monolithic (seamless) and slip resistant. Sheet vinyl (not tiles) or poured epoxy is acceptable. Coved bases are desirable and should be considered. Benches must be impervious to water and resistant to moderate heat and organic solvents, acids, alkalis, and decontamination chemicals. Chemically resistant plastic laminate, epoxy resin, and stainless steel are acceptable bench surfaces. Windows are permitted in BSL-3 labs but must be fixed and sealed. A decontamination method must be available in the facility, preferably within the lab. Approved decontamination methods include autoclaving and incineration. If waste is sent out of the lab for decontamination, it must be properly sealed and not transported in public corridors.

Air movement should be unidirectional, flowing into the lab from the clean areas and toward the dirty areas. Air must then be exhausted directly to the outside into areas with sunlight exposure. Rapid dilution of microorganisms on exhaust and the sun's ultraviolet rays make the use of high-efficiency particulate air (HEPA) filters optional, but when not employed, it is essential that the exhaust be located well away from air intakes and occupied areas. Alarmed, visual monitoring devices are recommended to keep an eye on airflow efficiency.

Biosafety Level Four

Because biosafety level four (BSL-4) labs are used for work with dangerous or exotic agents that pose a high risk of life-threatening disease, the design of BSL-4 labs expands significantly on BSL-3 requirements. Work requiring a BSL-4 lab is not generally encountered in a clinical environment. BSL-4 labs are usually seen in specialized research, often with animals.

Source: Adapted by Karen Mortland, president of Mortland Planning and Design, from the CDC.

addition to the microbiologic effects on air quality, a variety of chemicals may be used on a daily basis.) Consequently, labs can be hot, smelly places to work. When constructing a laboratory, organizations should consider the heating, ventilating, and air-conditioning (HVAC) unit to ensure the proper humidity, temperature control, and air exchanges in the lab. Pressure in relation to adjoining areas and corridors is also critical.

Temperature and Humidity

The laboratory houses a significant amount of heat-producing equipment. Organizations must ensure that temperature is controlled, is comfortable for staff, and is appropriate for the equipment.

Proper humidity must also be maintained in the laboratory environment. If a laboratory is too humid, the environment can foster the growth of bacteria and fungi. An environment without sufficient humidity levels can lead to static electricity issues.

Recommendations from agencies, such as the U.S. Department of Health and Human Services, include temperature ranges of 70°F, plus or minus five degrees, and a humidity range of 30%–55%.

Air Exchanges

There is some disagreement on how many air changes per hour (ACH) will ensure clean air in a laboratory. Both the AIA and the CDC weigh in on the issue, but their recommendations differ. The AIA recommends between 6 and 10 air changes, while the CDC supports 12 ACH for airborne droplet nuclei. "Twelve air changes remove approximately 99% of airborne particulates in 23 minutes. When only 6 air changes are employed, 46 minutes are required to accomplish the same task," says Mortland. Before deciding on the appropriate number of air changes, organizations should conduct their own risk assessment, consider the guidelines of the AIA, CDC, and other relevant organizations, and choose what is most appropriate for the particular laboratory.

In addition to air flow, it is critical that laboratory air not be recirculated to other areas of the health care organization, such as offices, corridors, or other laboratories. While air supply can come from other "clean" parts of the organization, such as offices or hallways, all laboratory exhaust must be vented outside. In addition, all openings in walls, ceilings, and floors for pipes, electrical conduit, and other components must be sealed to prevent air from leaking out of the lab and to maintain proper pressurization.

Storage

The amount of material that enters and exits a laboratory can be staggering. Add to it supplies, equipment, and new technology and a state-of-the-art lab can quickly have a storage issue. Designers should allow for plenty of storage within the lab to prevent laboratory personnel from storing things under desks, in front of fire exits, on chairs, and so forth. When designing venues for storage, such as shelving, organizations should consider ergonomic issues because some of the materials entering a laboratory may be heavy. As with other areas of the health care facility, organizations should limit the amount of stretching, lifting, bending, and reaching the staff must do.

One specific storage issue organizations will need to consider is refrigerated storage. Lab managers will need to decide between a walk-in cooler or standard refrigerators. Both of these types of coolers have their advantages. A walk-in cooler allows storage of large boxes, so laboratory personnel can unpack supply boxes when time permits. Refrigerators, however, require organization staff members to stop what they are doing to promptly unpack boxes. On the other hand, regular refrigerators are easy to move and, as the clinical laboratory morphs and changes over time, can be placed in other locations. Depending on the layout, a walk-in cooler may limit expansion options.

Acoustics

As previously mentioned, technology plays a significant role in the laboratory environment. While this technology can streamline processes, prevent errors, and ensure quality, it can also be noisy. Computer systems, automated equipment, and centrifuges all contribute to an environment with constant levels of white noise. Add phones, fax machines, and talking people and you have a symphony of noise. "One of the biggest complaints I hear from laboratory personnel is that the lab is too noisy," says Mortland.

One way to reduce noise in the lab is to use high sound-absorbance acoustical ceiling tiles. These should have a cleanable surface. While this can add expense to construction costs, the staff satisfaction and safety implications merit the expense. Other ways to reduce noise include the following:

Use cork. Cork is efficient at absorbing sound, and it is also naturally antimicrobial and antifungal. "Cork bulletin boards may be placed behind analyzers, refrigerators, and freezers to 'soak up' the noise this equipment produces. The partitions can easily be moved for equipment service and repair. They also have the capability of being cleanable, so they can meet the biosafety criteria," says Mortland.

Use recycled rubber flooring that is acoustically absorbent. "This eco-friendly flooring has the same acoustical properties as commercial carpeting yet meets the materials criteria for BSL-2 labs. It is naturally an excellent antifatigue flooring, has antislip qualities, absorbs vibration, does not promote bacterial or fungal growth, and is unaffected by heavy weights. As an additional bonus, in recent tests it has been found that paraffin does not stick to this flooring as it does to vinyl," Mortland says.

Use noise-absorbing wall boards. Similar to ceiling tiles, these wall boards should be completely cleanable.

Wrap conduits in sound-absorbing material. Noise from pipes, ducts, and pneumatic tube runs can be limited by wrapping these conduits with sound-absorbing material. Sound batting should be incorporated in the gypsum walls between rooms and, for optimum sound damping, should extend to the underside of the floor slab above. Sound from air handlers, elevators, dumbwaiters, and other building equipment can often be reduced by using vibration pads and flexible couplings that limit noise transmission.

Electronic sound masking. This is a relatively new and increasingly popular way to control noise in the workplace. Systems are designed to counter dominant background noises. Speakers are often placed above dropped ceilings and connected to a master control. Sound waves are introduced to the environment that effectively "cancel out" the target sound wave(s), rendering the space much quieter. "These systems have very effectively been used in large call centers and may work well in large, open lab designs. The dominant noise would be from a fairly constant source, such as refrigerators and freezers, and needs to be measured in the actual space to create the appropriate canceling noise," says Mortland.

Design for Flexibility

As with other areas of health care, clinical laboratories are changing all the time. "Most labs introduce some type of new equipment or technology every few months," Mortland says. Like other areas of the facility, organizations must design flexibility into the laboratory to accommodate new equipment and technology. Initial design should allow for smooth work flow so the staff is not tripping over things and can easily access their work and safety equipment. Design plans should also include ways the laboratory can be expanded or rearranged to accommodate new equipment, furniture, people, and supplies. Allowing an open footprint for the lab can aid in maintaining flexibility.

If a project involves the construction or renovation of a laboratory, it is important to involve laboratory management early in the planning process. The location of the laboratory, its equipment, and its ventilation system should all be discussed early in the planning process to prevent further headaches and expense later. Laboratory representation should continue throughout the design process because the needs of the laboratory change rapidly and new issues could arise before the facility is complete.

REFERENCE

1. Telephone interview with Karen Mortland, president of Mortland Planning and Design, Jun. 2005.

APPENDIX B:

Special Considerations for the Design of Pharmacies

PHARMACIES HAVE THEIR OWN set of design considerations, some of which are similar to those of laboratories. For example, pharmacies require cleanable surfaces, adequate storage, hands-free hand-wash sinks, eyewash stations, and other safety equipment.

Cleanrooms

The biggest aspect of pharmacy design is the IV preparation room, which is required to be a cleanroom. The International Standard Organization (ISO) defines a clean room as "a room in which the concentration of airborne particles is controlled, and which is constructed and used in a manner to minimize the introduction, generation, and retention of particles inside the room, and in which other relative parameters, such as temperature, humidity, and pressure, are controlled as necessary."[1]

Depending on the use, a pharmacy may be required by the United States Pharmacopoeia (USP) Chapter 797 to have one or more cleanrooms. (See Sidebar B-1). USP Chapter 797 governs the following aspects of the cleanroom:

- The size
- Air exchanges
- Particle counts
- Temperature
- Humidity

USP Standards are enforceable by the U.S. Food and Drug Administration (FDA) as well as are requirements of many state Boards of Pharmacy regulations. The Joint Commission also requires compliance with USP Chapter 797 (see *Joint Commission Perspectives*®, "Joint Commission to Survey Compliance with New USP-NF Chapter on Compounding Sterile Preparations," April 2004). During the planning stages of building design, organization pharmacists should research the USP Chapter 797 standards to determine the requirements for any necessary cleanrooms. For example, a small pharmacy may need a single cleanroom that allows for one individual in the room at any one time. A larger pharmacy may need to accommodate two to four individuals in the cleanroom. This will necessitate a larger room with greater air flow and exchanges. Other organizations will decide to use barrier isolators (also called "glove boxes") and will not need a cleanroom.

The USP is not the only organization that has specific standards for pharmacy facilities. Other entities requiring organizations to address specific issues in pharmacy design include the following:

SIDEBAR B-1.
USP Chapter 797

The USP is the official public standards-setting authority for all prescription and over-the-counter medicines, dietary supplements, and other health care products manufactured and sold in the United States. The USP sets standards for the quality of these products and works with health care providers to help them reach the standards.[2] USP Chapter 797 is the standard that deals with policies and practices for compounding sterile preparations. It took effect on January 1, 2004, and is the first official and enforceable requirement for compounding sterile preparations. By setting standards, requirements, and procedures for these preparations, USP Chapter 797 reduces the potential for contamination caused by an unclean environment, pharmacist error, lack of quality assurance, incorrect beyond-use dating, and other factors.

- International Standard Organization
- National Institute for Occupational Safety and Health (NIOSH)
- Occupational Safety and Health Administration (OSHA)
- FDA
- State Department of Health
- State Boards of Pharmacy

Pharmacists should familiarize themselves with all regulations before giving input on planning and design.

To ensure a properly designed cleanroom, organizations must control the concentration of airborne particles in that room. These particles can come from several sources, including the supply air, the individual(s) using the cleanroom, and the process being conducted in the cleanroom. Although USP Chapter 797 will dictate the specifics of cleanroom design, organizations should consider several overarching considerations. These considerations include the following:

Filtered supply air. Organizations can easily control the number of particles in the supplied air by using high-efficiency particulate air (HEPA) filters. As mentioned previously, most HEPA filters have a minimum efficiency of 99.97%.

Air exchanges. There is some discussion on the appropriate number of air exchanges necessary to maintain a clean environment. Depending on the volume of the room, the number of people in the room, and the type of work being conducted in the room, cleanrooms should have between 20 and 70 air exchanges per hour.[3]

Controlling infiltration. Particles from spaces adjacent to the cleanroom can be effectively managed by controlling the airflow direction so the air flows from the cleanroom to its adjacent space.[4] In most cases, this involves positively pressurizing the cleanroom. If an organization requires a cleanroom for preparing chemotherapy drugs, this room must be negatively pressurized with its own dedicated exhaust. While positively pressurized cleanrooms can be located next to negatively pressurized cleanrooms, they are not interchangeable.

One or more biosafety cabinets may be necessary. In most cases, these will be negatively pressurized.

Minimizing particles from cleanroom elements. Walls, floors, ceilings, and equipment can all release particles into the cleanroom. These can be reduced by using hard-surfaced, nonporous materials, such as polyvinyl panels, epoxy painted walls, and glass board ceilings.[4] Lighting should be sealed to prevent the release of particles, and the room should contain no ledges that could collect dust. Cleanroom surfaces and equipment must also be completely cleanable. Ceiling tiles should be sealed and walls should be laminated for easy cleaning.

Air filtration. Air within the cleanroom must be filtered with HEPA filters. Filtering must be done in conjunction with air exchanges to ensure a particle-free environment, rated ISO 7 or better.

Dedicated exhaust. Any exhaust from the cleanroom, including the exhaust from the centralized vacuums used to clean the cleanroom, must be exhausted through a dedicated source. Cleanroom exhaust from sterile preparation cleanrooms can share dedicated lines with other areas, if necessary. However, exhaust from cleanrooms used for chemotherapy preparation should be dedicated and vented to the outside. NIOSH has specific requirements in this area, and pharmacy departments should familiarize themselves with these requirements.

Before Using the Cleanroom

As with all other areas of a health care organization, the pharmacy should be thoroughly cleaned after construction and before occupancy. Cleanroom construction will expose the cleanroom to a significant amount of particulate matter.[5] Every surface of the cleanroom should be washed twice with a bactericidal, virucidal, phenolic, or a quaternary ammonium compound detergent. The third cleaning should involve the use of a diluted bleach solution. This three-step process will remove all foreign matter from the cleanroom.[5] All cleanrooms should be certified by a professional service to provide the specified level of particle levels before use.

Pharmacy Storage

Cleanroom design is not the only issue pharmacists and design teams should keep in mind when designing the pharmacy. For example, storage is a major consideration, as large quantities of chemicals, powders, medications, diluents, and so forth enter and must be stored in the pharmacy every day. Storage venues typically are cabinets or shelves. If not enough storage is available, pharmacists may need to get creative with storage and this may cause fire hazards. This can also negatively affect the airflow in the pharmacy. Typically, all products are cleaned prior to storage in the cleanroom to keep particle counts low.

Pharmacies in most health care organizations are busy spaces with several people moving about, and new supplies entering the room daily. Organizations may want to design a staging area in the pharmacy where staff members can temporarily store boxes of supplies until the staff has time to unload, stock the shelves, and break down the boxes. This can enhance the workflow of the pharmacy and prevent fire hazards. Because the ventilation systems and laminar flow airflow workbenches (in other words, "hoods") generate a tremendous amount of noise, it is important that there be a fire alarm in the cleanroom so staff working in the room can hear it.

Gaining Pharmacy Input Early

Because of the complex nature of cleanroom design, as well as the specific requirements of USP 797, a pharmacy cannot be placed just anywhere in an organization. Besides the IV preparation room or cleanroom, many new pharmacies are including sophisticated computer technology and automation such as dispensing robotics, bar code packaging machines, and other equipment that are designed to reduce medication errors but take considerable space in the pharmacy. Organizations that think about pharmacy location, position, and layout as an afterthought will run into tremendous problems and expense later in the project. The pharmacy department needs to be involved in the design process right up front, and collaboration between the pharmacy department, architects, and engineers should continue throughout the entire planning, design, and construction process. Although every organization's needs are different, the case study on pages 132–133 explains one organization's experience in planning, designing, and constructing a pharmacy.

Case Study B-1. Involving the Pharmacy Early Ensures Appropriate Design

The University of Utah Hospitals and Clinics' Experience in Designing New Pharmacies

As part of a recent construction project, the University of Utah Hospitals and Clinics, located in Salt Lake City, built three new pharmacies and remodeled one existing pharmacy. "We recently opened a new cancer hospital, orthopedic hospital, and ambulatory cancer infusion center. Each of these facilities had a new pharmacy and then we remodeled the central pharmacy to accommodate all the new technology associated with these new facilities," says Jim Jorgenson, administrative director for pharmacy and associate dean of pharmacy for the University of Utah. "Our goals in this process were to improve patient and staff safety and enhance operational efficiency."

Early Involvement of the Pharmacy

The planning and design process began five years ago, and the pharmacy department was involved in the planning stage up front. "Typically, architects have a preconceived notion about where the pharmacy should go. Unfortunately, their assumptions are usually wrong. Pharmacies cannot be crammed into leftover space. This leads to incorrect placement, insufficient space, and the inability to expand with new technology. In addition, the requirements of NIOSH and the USP are not considered," Jorgenson says.

Unlike some organizations, the University of Utah involved pharmacists in the planning process right away. Through a series of meetings, the pharmacy department educated senior leadership and the design team on the considerations relevant to pharmacy design. Pharmacy management provided and explained the relevant standards and brought in architects to the pharmacy to watch current operations. "We also conducted a failure modes and effects analysis on the pharmacy to identify possible problem issues that needed to be addressed in design. In addition, we asked the Institute of Safe Medication Practices (ISMP) to come in and conduct its own risk analysis," states Jorgenson.

Design Strategies

As a result of its research and planning efforts, the University of Utah focused on several issues during pharmacy design.

Proper air handling. The organization ensured that all contaminated exhaust was vented to the outside, that proper humidity and temperature were controlled within the pharmacy, and that the number of air exchanges was appropriate for the use of the facility. "In addition, we designed the cleanrooms so that they could be changed from positive to negative pressure environments without too much expense. This allowed some flexibility for further growth and change," says Jorgenson.

Hand-wash sinks. The organization took special care to ensure that all hand-wash sinks and eyewash stations were properly placed to be easily accessible and to meet USP standards. Hand-wash sinks should also be hands free.

Pharmaceutical delivery. Because of the size of the organization, significant time could be spent delivering medications to other pharmacies or nursing units. To address this issue, the University of Utah installed a tube system that allowed medications to be easily transferred between locations.

Work flow. To ensure efficient work flow in the pharmacy, the organization considered door placement, an entry point for supplies and medications, data entry positions, and storage. "We wanted to make sure that any data entry activities took place in a secluded, quiet area so as to ensure an uninterrupted environment. This helps increase efficiency, improve work flow, and prevent mistakes," Jorgenson says. Doors might also need to be automatic to allow for deliveries on carts.

Storage. The organization incorporated both fixed storage (shelving units) and automated carousels into the pharmacy. The organization considered how much storage was necessary, based on current inventory and potential inventory issues. "We also examined the refrigerator/freezer capacity we needed and incorporated that into the design," states Jorgenson.

Standardization. Because the organization was constructing three new pharmacies and renovating an existing one, it had the opportunity to stan-

Continued on page 133

Continued from page 132

dardize the equipment, design, and work flow of the facilities. This allowed staff members to move between the facilities and not take time familiarizing themselves with layout and equipment.

During Construction

The University of Utah assigned a construction supervisor to be in charge of the pharmacy construction aspect of the building project. Pharmacy leaders met daily with this supervisor to review progress and discuss any issues. "We were in constant communication, which helped us identify and address issues early," says Jorgenson. "It was a tremendous help to have the ear and attention of a dedicated construction manager linked to the entire design and construction team."

Measuring Success

To measure the success of its new design, the University of Utah measured several things, including the following:

- Medication errors
- Turnaround time
- Stock outs
- Inventory turns
- Efficiency

"We are currently measuring these elements, and are pleased with the progress. We are looking to further improve, but the design of the pharmacies has definitely made a difference," Jorgenson says.

Lessons Learned

"The biggest lesson we learned in this process is the importance of detailed and advanced planning. While you don't need to know all the details up front, it is important to have a strategic plan for the pharmacy and know how you are going to operationalize that plan," states Jorgenson. Constant communication with architects, organization leaders, and construction teams helped the University design standardized, integrated, efficient pharmacies that preserve staff and patient safety.

CASE AT A GLANCE

■ Main challenge
To design a series of pharmacies that enhanced staff and patient safety while maintaining efficiency.

■ Issues
The design of pharmacies must meet several regulations, including those of NIOSH and the USP. Pharmacy managers must be involved early in the planning and design process to ensure that all regulations are met.

■ Solutions
By educating the design team and senior leadership on the needs of the pharmacy, actively participating in planning, design, and construction efforts, and maintaining constant communication with the design and construction teams, the university was able to design appropriate, safe, and efficient facilities.

■ Outcomes
All four of the organization's pharmacies are standardized, integrated, and effectively address air flow, storage, and infection control issues.

REFERENCES

1. ISO 14644.1999. Cleanrooms and associated controlled environments.

2. United States Pharmocopeia: *About USP—An Overview.* http://www.usp.org/aboutUSP/ (accessed Jun. 30, 2005).

3. Telephone interview with Bruce Harrison, clinical pharmacy specialist. Veterans Affairs Medical Center, St. Louis, May 2005.

4. Zhang J.: Understanding pharmaceutical cleanroom design. *ASHRAE Journal* pp. 29–33, Sep. 2004.

5 Kastango E., DeMarco S.: Pharmacy cleanroom project management considerations: An experienced-based perspective. *International Journal of Pharmaceutical Compounding* 5: May/Jun. 2001.

INDEX

Note: The page numbers in this index are coded as follows: n refers to note. **BOLD** type indicates **Case Study** or **Sidebar**

A

B

C

G

H

I

J

L

M

N

O

P

R

S

T

U

V

W